The Atkins Diet and Philosophy

Popular Culture and Philosophy™
Series Editor: William Irwin

Volume 1
Seinfeld and Philosophy: A Book about Everything and Nothing (2000) Edited by William Irwin

Volume 2
The Simpsons and Philosophy: The D'oh! of Homer (2001) Edited by William Irwin, Mark T. Conard, and Aeon J. Skoble

Volume 3
The Matrix and Philosophy: Welcome to the Desert of the Real (2002) Edited by William Irwin

Volume 4
Buffy the Vampire Slayer and Philosophy: Fear and Trembling in Sunnydale (2003) Edited by James B. South

Volume 5
The Lord of the Rings and Philosophy: One Book to Rule Them All (2003) Edited by Gregory Bassham and Eric Bronson

Volume 6
Baseball and Philosophy: Thinking Outside the Batter's Box (2004) Edited by Eric Bronson

Volume 7
The Sopranos and Philosophy: I Kill Therefore I Am (2004) Edited by Richard Greene and Peter Vernezze

Volume 8
Woody Allen and Philosophy: You Mean My Whole Fallacy Is Wrong? (2004) Edited by Mark T. Conard and Aeon J. Skoble

Volume 9
Harry Potter and Philosophy: If Aristotle Ran Hogwarts (2004) Edited by David Baggett and Shawn E. Klein

Volume 10
Mel Gibson's Passion and Philosophy: The Cross, the Questions, the Controversy (2004) Edited by Jorge J.E. Gracia

Volume 11
More Matrix and Philosophy: Revolutions and Reloaded Decoded (2005) Edited by William Irwin

Volume 12
Star Wars and Philosophy (2005) Edited by Jason T. Eberl and Kevin S. Decker

Volume 13
Superheroes and Philosophy (2005) Edited by Tom Morris and Matt Morris

Volume 14
The Atkins Diet and Philosophy: Chewing the Fat with Kant and Nietzsche (2005) Edited by Lisa Heldke, Kerri Mommer, and Cynthia Pineo

Volume 15
The Chronicles of Narnia and Philosophy: The Lion, the Witch, and the Worldview (2005) Edited by Gregory Bassham and Jerry L. Walls

In Preparation:

Hip Hop and Philosophy: Rhyme 2 Reason (2005) Edited by Derrick Darby and Tommie Shelby

Bob Dylan and Philosophy (2006) Edited by Carl Porter and Peter Vernezze

Monty Python and Philosophy: Nudge Nudge, Think Think (2006) Edited by Gary L. Hardcastle and George A. Reisch

Popular Culture and Philosophy™

The Atkins Diet and Philosophy

Chewing the Fat with Kant and Nietzsche

Edited by
LISA HELDKE, KERRI MOMMER,
and CYNTHIA PINEO

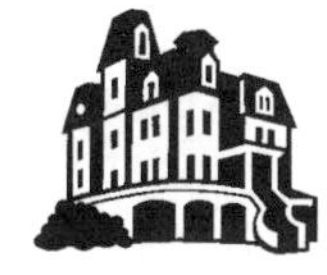

OPEN COURT
Chicago and La Salle, Illinois

Volume 14 in the series, Popular Culture and Philosophy™

To order books from Open Court, call toll-free 1-800-815-2280, or visit www.opencourtbooks.com.

Open Court Publishing Company is a division of Carus Publishing Company.

First printing 2005

Printed and bound in the United States of America.

Library of Congress Cataloging-in-Publication Data

The Atkins diet and philosophy : chewing the fat with Kant and Nietzsche / edited by Lisa Heldke, Kerri Mommer, and Cynthia Pineois.
p. cm. – (Popular culture and philosophy ; v. 14)
Includes bibliographical references and index.
ISBN-13: 978-0-8126-9584-7 (trade pbk. : alk. paper)
ISBN-10: 0-8126-9584-4 (trade pbk. : alk. paper)
1. Reducing diets. I. Heldke, Lisa M. (Lisa Maree), 1960- . II. Mommer, Kerri, 1958 - . III. Pineo, Cynthia, 1971- . IV. Series.
RM222.2.A837 2005
613.2'5—dc22 2005018931

To our sweeties and honeypies:

David and Arlo

Veronica, Reggie, and Mike

Contents

Part 3: Carbohydrates

Part 4: Vitamins and Minerals

Part 5: Unlimited Noncaloric Beverages

Acknowledgments

This book would not have been possible without our authors, who labored long and hard to create the tasty contributions you are about to enjoy. This all goes to show that too many cooks don't spoil the broth. Thanks also go to David Ramsay Steele and Bill Irwin for their support and enthusiasm and to Carolyn Madia Gray for getting the word out.

In(tro)duction: Setting the Table

Ever since Plato proposed a diet of roasted meats for his guardians while on campaign (they're easy to prepare, you don't have to carry any cooking pots, and cleanup is a breeze!),[1] the subject of our diet—what we eat, and why—has hovered on the edges of philosophers' attention. Once in a while, it has emerged into a full-blown discussion, as in Nietzsche's book *Ecce Homo,* which includes a lengthy disquisition on his own dietary choices. But most of what philosophers have had to say about diet could be written on small Post-it Notes. (Care for an example? Did you know that it was a philosopher who first said "You are what you eat"? Ludwig Feuerbach made the observation in 1850.[2] By the way, the expression is a lot catchier in the original German: "Der Mensch ist was er isst.")

In point of fact, there is no shortage of philosophically relevant issues involving food—growing it, distributing it, preparing it, eating it, and then sending it on to its next task. And some philosophers have long been deeply engaged in examining some of these issues, including sociopolitical issues about hunger and justice and ethical issues about vegetarianism. The

---

[1] Plato, *Republic,* Book 3, translated by Benjamin Jowett, available online at Classic Reader website, http://www.classicreader.com/read.php/sid.8/bookid.1788/sec.24/.

[2] Feuerbach makes the comment in a discussion of the work of physiologist Jacob Moleschott, entitled "The Natural Sciences and the Revolution." Feuerbach goes on to observe, "Now we know, on scientific grounds, what the masses know from long experience, that eating and drinking hold together body and soul, that the searched-for bond is nutrition." Quoted in Marx Wartofsky, *Feuerbach* (Cambridge: Cambridge University Press, 1977), p. 414.

past fifteen years have witnessed the emergence of even more philosophical interest in food, including topics ranging from environmental ethics (biotechnology, factory farming) to aesthetics (taste, disgust) to epistemology and metaphysics (cooking as theory making, food and personhood). In case the present volume whets your appetite for more, we've included a brief bibliography of historical and contemporary works in the philosophy of food.

But while philosophers do at least sometimes talk about food, and even about our diet, perhaps only one philosopher—Richard Watson—has directly taken on the topic of diet*ing*—that is, a program of eating designed to lose weight. But his *Philosopher's Diet* is really interested in telling his readers *how* to lose weight—in a reflective, philosophical way, of course.[3] Unlike Richard Watson, we don't really want to diet; we just want to *think* about dieting. And what better way to bring the philosophical reflection on dieting down to gut level, than a collection of ruminations on one of the most significant diet movements of our age—the Atkins Diet?

Oh, not that there haven't been a few skeptics—initially, at least. In conversations at philosophy conferences, for instance, the most common reaction we received, when we reported that Open Court was going to publish a book on the Atkins Diet and philosophy, was barking laughter. But once listeners realized we weren't kidding, they'd ponder, silently, for a few minutes, and then perform a conceptual one-eighty. "You know, that's not such a crazy idea after all. In fact, *I* can think of a few things I'd like to say about that topic—especially after the lunch I just endured/enjoyed with my colleague who isn't/is on the Atkins/South Beach/NeanderThin diet."

This volume collects sixteen essays by contributors who chew on the diet from a number of philosophical angles and a variety of personal perspectives. Here, you can sample essays written by practitioners of the Atkins Diet or one of its low-carb cousins; by people who are not on the diet; and by people who choose to keep mum about their own current relationships to carbohydrates. (We made an editorial decision to respect their right to remain silent on the matter of whether or not sliced

[3] Richard A. Watson, *The Philosopher's Diet: How to Lose Weight and Change the World* (Boston: Godine, 1999).

bread *is* the greatest thing since, well, since unsliced bread.) Not only do the writers collected here represent a range of personal eating practices; they also represent a considerable diversity of philosophical perspectives. Here you'll find essays using the Atkins Diet to illustrate ideas from such historically important philosophers as Kant, Hume, Nietzsche, Marx, and Dewey. But you'll also find essays that examine the diet from the perspective of contemporary environmental philosophy, feminist philosophy, critical race theory, philosophy of science, and pragmatism (to mention just a few of the philosophical approaches employed). Some of the essays use Atkins to illuminate philosophy, others use philosophy to illuminate Atkins, and some do a little of both. All of the essays invite you to think—more carefully, perhaps, than you usually do—about *why* you eat what you choose to eat. They're not here to tell you what to think—or what to eat, for that matter. But that doesn't mean they aren't going to give you plenty of ideas to digest—at least some of which might leave you feeling bit queasy. Hopefully some of them will also make you laugh—which, as we all know, is a great digestive aid.

* * * * *

Why the *Atkins* Diet and philosophy rather than some other diet? First, the Atkins Diet has shown more longevity than most diets, having first reached popularity over three decades ago. It cannot be dismissed as a fad—even though some of the more bizarre comestibles it has inspired might deserve that moniker. (Does anyone really believe cinnamon-flavored pork rinds are here to stay?) Second, the eating plan that Atkins advocates is a radical departure from both traditional "balanced diet" plans (such as Weight Watchers or Jenny Craig) and low-fat diets. In fact, because the Atkins eating plan seems so counterintuitive, and since it seems to fly in the face of much current expert opinion, this diet raises chewy philosophical questions about how to decide the best way to eat, how to decide what to believe, and how to decide who to believe about dietary matters.

* * * * *

Okay, then, why the Atkins Diet and *philosophy?* For centuries, philosophy was regarded as the "queen of the sciences." As such, it had a tendency—annoying or utterly warranted, depending upon your perspective—to stick its nose in everywhere, and to pronounce on everything. After all, it was the queen; it had a responsibility to make meta-pronouncements! Today, many philosophers are less likely to address the discipline as Your Highness, but we still believe that *reflective, theoretical* questions surround every form of intellectual inquiry, and that these questions can and ought to be examined, both by people within those disciplines and by philosophers.

* * * * *

Is there something Pavlovian about the fact that mentioning the topics of food and philosophy together will invariably trigger the bad pun response in people? No, we mean it; *really* bad puns. Puns far worse than the run-of-the-mill bad puns that often serve as subtitles for the Popular Culture and Philosophy series. You don't believe us, eh? (Or does that scowl on your face just mean you're too busy thinking up your own bad pun to respond?) Consider, if you will, some of the subtitles that were found littering the table after an editorial meeting (amidst the no-carb energy bar wrappers and the fragment of a bagel that someone had failed to fully conceal in a paper napkin):

Thus Steak Zarathustra
The Seamy Underbelly of Philosophy
Twilight of the Carbos
Meataphysical Ruminations
The Carbegorical Imperative
Sinking Your Teeth into the War on Carbs
Steak and Eggheads
Driving a Steak through Carbs
Meaty Issues
Fleshing Out the Dry Bones of . . .
Hamming It Up . . .

(The last two were obviously so bad that the brainstormer didn't bother to finish the thought.)

Sit back, get comfortable, and grab your favorite low-carb treat, be it chicken satay with peanut dipping sauce, sugar-free mocha ricotta crème, spicy pork rinds with guacamole, or a modest handful of chili-roasted macadamia nuts, along with a cup of decaf coffee with heavy cream or a tall, cool glass of lemonade (made with Splenda® of course). Then you'll be ready to eat, drink (or read, think), and be merry, for tomorrow you shall diet.

Part 1

Protein

(Personal Choice and Action)

1

Cutting the Conceptual Carbs: Dewey as Dietician, Atkins as Pragmatist

RANDALL E. AUXIER

Dr. Atkins has trimmed our waistlines, changed our way of looking at the familiar processes of the human body, and certainly taken our money. One would think this would be enough of an achievement for one lifetime. But I wonder if we might not squeeze a bit more from his "revolution" than even he imagined. Maybe, just maybe, Atkins has hit upon something that can help us with another epidemic. I think so, at least. I want to use something I learned from Dr. Atkins to explain something I think everyone ought to grasp, which is the philosophy of pragmatism.

Doubtful Beginnings

The philosophy of pragmatism has made a marked difference in the domain of human thinking, enjoying a lengthy heyday from the 1890s up through the early 1950s, and enjoying a new resurgence of attention and influence in the last two decades. Philosophical pragmatism does not tell us what we should *do*; rather, it gives us some norms and rules for our *thinking* (of course thinking is doing *something*, but let's not quibble over details just yet). Perhaps the most important pragmatist was John Dewey (1859–1952), who managed to write exactly ten times as many books as you have time to read, and to smoke cigarettes every day of his adult life and still live to be ninety-two. A man like that commands respect. Just thinking about it makes me want a cigarette. But I bring him up here not because I want a cigarette, although I do (with the help of

Dewey's philosophy I quit smoking in 1988—and again in 1996 and 2002), but because Dewey knew something that will help us understand *why* the Atkins Diet works, which is where I want to start this story, before moving to what Atkins can teach us about pragmatism.

Dr. Atkins himself explains the physiological reasons why his diet works well enough,[1] but I am in pursuit of something a little more general than that. I'm looking for a kind of "self-knowledge," a philosophical reflection upon why the diet works, and in so doing, with your indulgence, I need to start with why it worked *for me*.

Pragmatists insist on restricting inquiry to "genuine doubt," as distinct from the over-used "hyperbolic doubt" employed by René Descartes and his followers. Hyperbolic or exaggerated doubt is a popular method in very abstract types of philosophies, doubt of sort that goes beyond what is inspired by pressing problems and ordinary curiosity. Pragmatists don't care for it. Hyperbolic doubt won't bring you any toilet paper when you're stranded. And obviously life is short and we haven't got time to doubt everything; as with friends, pick your doubts carefully. So, returning to Atkins, part of what causes this to be a "genuine doubt" for me is that I have had a personal stake in it. I don't doubt that the Atkins Diet works for a lot of people, but I did doubt that I fully understood why. Now I think I get part of the reason.

Kitchen Confessions of a Pragmatist

First, the ugly story of success: While I was not fat in 2001, I had about twenty extra pounds, and entering midlife I knew I was not healthy. Every time I quit smoking I would pick up five or seven pounds, for example, and somehow not drop them again when I started back, which seems grossly unfair. I mean, if there were a *benevolent* God or *any* justice in the universe, at the very least we should be trim from destroying our lungs. But no. I had actually tried a low-fat diet in the fall of that year—which put ten more pounds on me, thank you very

[1] Robert C. Atkins, *Dr. Atkins' New Diet Revolution*, revised edition (New York: Avon, 2002), Part 1, pp. 3–104.

much. Without realizing it or understanding it, I was making up for the loss of protein and fat in my diet by consuming more carbs, and as it turns out, I am particularly susceptible to carbs—adult-onset diabetes runs in the family. So I went on the Atkins Diet in February of 2002 and lost twenty pounds in short order during Induction. I stayed on Induction until June of that year, and then went on the OWL program (ongoing weight loss), gradually losing another fifteen pounds by August of 2004, achieving my goal weight in that month. I celebrated with a cigarette, but only one.

All of the things Dr. Atkins promised came to pass in my case. No more sugar crashes after meals (the blood sugar yo-yo), more energy; I felt better, and I was able to negotiate this diet in such a way as to make it into a sustainable lifestyle. As Atkins promised, I do take great delight in the foods I get to eat, and the only things I really miss are bread and pasta. But now I can occasionally nibble a crust, although negotiating the "maintenance" part of the diet has been a little trickier than I thought—I like wine a little too much, I think, but then, so did Jesus according to some of his ancient critics. Unlike Jesus I have to *pay* for mine, but all things considered, I wouldn't trade places with Jesus just for the free wine. Yes, yes, good for you, Auxier, whoop-de-doo, you and Jesus are skinny. As a matter of fact, I am happier too, although I firmly suspect this has to do with having deeply internalized a bit of "junkthought" regarding how I *ought* to look, perhaps from consuming too many television images for thirty years. But there is no denying that this mindless and ironic cult of youth we live in likes to see a flat stomach, while almost 65 percent of us are overweight and over 30 percent are obese.[2] Countering this obsession with skeletal supermodels, I have noticed how the models in the pictures at Wal-Mart's clothing department are almost all pretty stout these days, and the shirts that we used to call "extra-large" we now call "medium." It's disturbing to me when Wal-Mart becomes a more reliable barometer of reality than television. But I guess their marketing people have been to Wal-Mart, on occasion, and have noticed who is shopping there. The underwear aisle is enough to turn anyone to Atkins.

---

[2] Robert C. Atkins, *Atkins for Life* (New York: St. Martin's Press, 2003), p. ix.

"Habits and Habitats"

Now my conjecture is that Atkins works not only because it has a sound physiological basis, but also because it taps into our already established habits, and here is where Dewey can be our dietician. Dewey is one of only a few major Western moral philosophers, along with David Hume (1711–1776) and Aristotle (384–322 B.C.E.), who sees "habit" as the Archimedean point of the good life. Dewey says:

> The difficulty in the way of attaining and maintaining practical wisdom is the urgency of immediate impulse and desire which swell and swell until they crowd out all thought of remote and comprehensive goods. The conflict is a real one and is at the heart of many of our more serious struggles and lapses. In the main, solution is found in utilizing all possible occasions, when we are not in the presence of conflicting desires, to cultivate interest in those goods which we do approve in our calm moments of reflection. . . . There are many times when the cultivation of these interests meets with no strong obstacle. The habits which are built up and reenforced under such conditions are the best bulwarks against weakness and surrender in the moments when the reflective or "true" good conflicts with that set up by temporary and intense desire.[3]

Dewey never won any prizes for writing, but the message is clear enough. If you want to live wisely and well, form good habits when you are *not* in the throes of desire. As Bill Clinton will eagerly testify, you don't do your best decision-making in amorous moments, especially relative to the long-term values you embrace when she isn't around. Those good habits rehearsed and enacted by the calm heart and sated stomach are what will best sustain you when you come to a difficult moment of choice. We could do worse than to make Dewey our dietician. Dr. Atkins supplements our choice by pointing out that you can have much of what you *want* in answer to those very foreseeable crises, a steak for the black eye of desire. Make a few good choices about *how* to gratify your desires, according to a few time-proven, long-term principles, get into the habit of making those choices, and the short-term crisis of desire can be weathered.

---

[3] John Dewey, *The Later Works, 1925–1953, Volume 7: Ethics, 1932* (Carbondale: Southern Illinois University Press, 1985), p. 208.

Before moving to a more thorough discussion of pragmatism with Atkins as our guide, I think it should be pointed out that people (such as I) who do not have any special affinity for sugar have a far easier beast to tame than do those for whom sugar is the very *bête noire.* My special carbo-weakness was for bread and pasta, but luckily I cared little for potatoes, corn, or anything with sugar in it. The alteration of my habits led me away from Italian restaurants (a great loss) and required me to tread carefully in Mexican places, and I was obliged to throw out about twenty of my favorite recipes, since (contrary to the claims of Robert and Veronica Atkins) they never have and never will make edible pasta out of soy. I now realize I will probably never cook or order pasta again, and that I am doomed to scour Mexican menus for odd words like *ceviche* and Italian ones for *pesche.* That is a long-term sacrifice that I seem to be able (so far) to maintain. My only alternative to the sacrifice would be exercise, and I know myself better than to imagine that I will do something that resolutely refuses to become a habit. And from this moment of self-honesty a general point emerges, which is that Atkins or any other diet (or lifestyle) really has to be interpreted relative to the individual problem one faces, and then applied pragmatically to *that* problem. My unscientific guess is that people who already don't care for sugar and potatoes have the best luck with Atkins, since the habits associated with the diet are, for them, easily acquired. Also, I would suppose, again unscientifically (I have read the controversies and can form no opinion), that people who are fighting cholesterol, heart problems, and high blood pressure might do better on a low-fat, low-sodium diet than on Atkins. Meanwhile, it would seem that people whose main trouble is avoiding adult-onset diabetes will likely derive more benefit from finding their own way of doing Atkins, but in all cases, the task is one of modifying habits in ways that are maintainable both in the short and long term.

Atkins encourages us without surcease to adopt the sorts of habits that can be sustained; he tells us that we cannot seriously expect to stay on a diet under whose draconian reign we become as peasants waif and wan. But what is a habit anyway? Dewey says:

> [W]e need a word to express the kind of human activity which is influenced by prior activity and in that sense acquired; which

> contains within itself a certain ordering or systematization of minor elements of action; which is projective and dynamic in quality, ready for overt manifestation; and which is operative in some subdued subordinate form even when not obviously dominating activity. Habit even in its ordinary usage comes nearer to denoting these facts than any other word.[4]

Reading Dewey is like eating oatmeal, but sometimes there is a raisin mixed in. Not this time, I grant. On that note I would also add that oatmeal is too high in carbs, but raisins are worse by far. But a habit, in less mushy language, is a way we carry our personal histories around with us as both a spring to and an inhibitor of present and future action. If you know, for example, that the last two times you started smoking again were due to a weak moment at a convenience-store counter, it might be best to take notice of this and pay for your gas with a credit card from the safety of the pump. I haven't seen the inside of a convenience store since, well, since I last quit smoking. That is not an accident. That is a matter of understanding habits, in Dewey's sense. In this way Dewey supplements our understanding of why the Atkins Diet works for so many people, but we might do better to be aware that a Deweyan diet urges us to adapt the generalizations to the problem, not the problem to the pre-existing generalizations. Atkins never suggested otherwise, of course, but his critics like to overlook his copious qualifying statements.

Peirce's Pragmatic Propadeutic: Piercings and Pigmented Pictures

Now perhaps we are in a position to discover what Dr. Atkins teaches us that he never meant to—about philosophy and how to think.

For as long as the word "pragmatic" has been a part of our common tongue, it has carried both positive and negative associations. Other words like "shrewd," or "ambitious," or even "creative" (as in "creative accounting") have had similar careers. Such delightful words enable one to speak out of both sides of one's mouth (regardless of what one is putting into it). And per-

---

[4] John Dewey, *The Middle Works, 1899–1924, Volume 14: Human Nature and Conduct, 1922* (Carbondale: Southern Illinois University Press, 1983), p. 31.

haps this delectable ambiguity will seem even tastier when I say that Robert Atkins was a pragmatist. Indeed, I can imagine precious few examples of pragmatism more complete than his diet, and even fewer public philosophers of the present generation who more thoroughly *embody* (and I mean that literally) the ideals of pragmatism. But what, pray tell, is pragmatism?

The eccentric American philosopher and mathematician Charles S. Peirce (1839–1914),[5] is traditionally known as the founder of "pragmatism." But this maven of mental calisthenics was more concerned for the health of our thinking than for the health of our bodies, and in this regard he recommended a strict mental diet and a rigorous exercise program. Do not leap to conclusions: Peirce did not despise bodies, especially feminine ones, being rumored to have possessed a large collection of Victorian pornography,[6] but his pragmatism focused more upon getting our thinking in shape, in hopes that bodily excellence might follow rather than the converse. Here is his master principle, called "the pragmatic maxim":

> Consider what effects, which might conceivably have practical bearings, we conceive the objects of our conception to have. Then, our conception of these effects is the whole of our conception of the object.[7]

The exercise here available for the reader should be obvious, since a more tortured bit of prose is scarcely imaginable (and I have made a point of preserving Peirce's unfathomable punctuation). Subsequent generations of professors have grown flaccid

---

[5] The name is pronounced "purse," something your mother would have carried; not "pierce," a popular anatomical modification your teenaged son or daughter is probably hiding from you.

[6] The last thing I want to do is contribute more grist for the rumor mill surrounding the unfortunate Peirce, but there is more than enough documented muck and slime to satisfy any reader of the *National Enquirer*. I can scarcely damage Peirce's character more than he did himself. See the biography by Joseph Brent, *Charles Sanders Peirce: A Life* (Bloomington: Indiana University Press, 1993), and also Brent's story of his duels with the Harvard community that was trying to bury the ugly truth: http://members.door.net/arisbe/menu/library/aboutcsp/brent/singular.htm.

[7] C.S. Peirce, *The Writings of Charles S. Peirce: A Chronological Edition* (Bloomington: Indiana University Press, 1986), Volume 3, p. 266.

in their armchairs while exercising their brains on these two sentences. It is a complete diet for the mind. The economy of it is also impressive; anyone can afford the time to read these two sentences, but only the few have the leisure to ponder their meanings. To save you time, let me summarize what these sentences might mean, bypassing the issue of what they actually *do* mean. Here are eight steps in a recipe to help you understand Peirce's pragmatic maxim, in approximately the order you would use them:

1. When you think, you are thinking *about* something (unless you are a politician).
2. Ask yourself: "How should I *define* the thing I'm thinking about; in other words, what are its characteristics and limits?"
3. It turns out that whatever you are thinking about has effects on the world (whether you like it or not), so just think of those effects.
4. Now try thinking of your thing in two different ways (or more, but not right now since you're a beginner).
5. Take stock of the practical consequences that follow from thinking about it first one way, then the other.
6. If there's no difference, you're thinking of the same thing.
7. If there's a difference, you're thinking of two different things.
8. The list of the differences is what you use to separate the thing you're thinking about from other things you're *not* thinking about, but aren't currently sure you aren't thinking about.

For example, let's begin with a situation that inspires genuine doubt in us, recalling that pragmatists have no patience for any other kind of doubt. As a test, if the doubt doesn't at least get you up off the couch, it probably isn't worth the trouble. Genuine doubt is the trigger of thinking, according to pragmatists; according to them, we *only* think when we are in doubt. The rest of the time, we are pretty happy. Let's say you are thinking: "I wonder if my teenaged daughter has a tattoo or a piercing?" You are thinking *about* something here, but how to define it? What is the crux of the concern? Is it the idea that she might have pierced her body with steel somewhere, carelessly bleeding your family's blood all over some strange floor for no reason better than to defy your wishes and impress her friends? Or is it that some biker who goes by the name of Snake has seen (and marked) parts of her body that you used to wash but now cannot remember? It would be wise to sort this out before acting on the doubt.

Let us see if the pragmatic maxim helps us clarify our thinking. First let us define the concern. Our pragmatic guide might inquire: Does it make a practical difference if it is a piercing or a tattoo? Of course; they are different. For instance, piercings generally grow back together on their own. Tattoos are expensive to remove. (Apparently time does not heal *all* wounds.) But this difference seems not to settle the doubt that created the question. Were you really worried about the medical expense of removing a tattoo when she is forty and realizes how ridiculous she looks? No. This was not the concern. This difference does not make a difference, unless you intend to be paying her medical expenses when she wakes up to the harsh realities of sagging flesh in mid-life, that is, when she discovers the wonders of Dr. Atkins. The list of these differences between piercings and tattoos will make it clear that for all practical purposes they are the same idea, in this context, and you need to seek another way of looking at your idea.

What *were* you thinking about? We may proceed upon these lines until you have landed upon the "concept" that corresponds serviceably to your initial doubt, and until we have traced out all the variations in consequences that can be helpful, and all that lies beyond this betokens a different situation, a different doubt. For example, you may recognize that, following the line of implications, your *real* concern is about having your wishes defied by your daughter, if you are a particularly egocentric parent. Or perhaps you are really less worried about marks and piercings than about the company she is keeping (Snake and his buddies), and the consequences that might follow from this. Whatever the case, your *thinking* is aided by pursuing the noble eightfold path above, and even if you have no idea what you should *do*, at least you know what you are thinking about. A side benefit of the pragmatic method is that, over time, it would put psychologists out of business—but it would be a bonanza for anyone with a workable idea for a diet.

Conceptual Carbs: An Induction Program

If we use Dr. Atkins to help us grasp pragmatism, we can imagine that thinking a thought is sort of like consuming a morsel, and while certain thoughts are perhaps high in mental fat, some others might be high in conceptual carbohydrates. As Atkins teaches us, "losing weight is not a matter of counting calories; it is a matter of eating food your body is able to handle."[8] Analogously, conceptual gluttony is not our main problem. Of course there are only so many hours in the day, and we probably ought not spend all of them thinking. But as with eating, we all have to think, so the question of being mentally fit and trim is really more about what we think, not how much. So, pragmatically speaking, let us not waste our effort counting "mental calories."

Also we should not go on mental starvation diets—drinking or taking recreational drugs, meditating, or seeking political office—just to keep us from having to think. Nay, that would be neither pragmatic nor practical. So release your fantasies about trying to "be in the moment," or any of those other faddish ways of *not* thinking. Think with gusto, just like Dr. Atkins standing behind his "huge table heaped with food"—in this case, food for thought.[9] Think away. But on the other side, Atkins teaches us to be wary of overly processed ideas and junkthoughts, these "high-sugar horrors."[10] Preparing to change the way we think involves not mere mind games; this is about your long-term happiness. Do not be a profligate thinker, deconstructing every idea that hitches a ride in your cortex; stop playing dialectical games with yourself, playing Plato (whose name apparently meant, in the vernacular, "fatty") to your own Socrates (who was also far too stout to run from Marathon to Athens). And do not by any means go to the university philosophers, those *maître d's* of minced logic, a veritable McDonald's of mind, where thoughts are analyzed into such tiny fragments that even their mothers can no longer recognize them, and then recombined into monstrously unhealthy tidbits of intellectual trivia. No Mental McDonald's for the aspiring pragmatist. Indeed these

[8] Atkins, *New Diet Revolution*, p. 11.

[9] *Ibid.*, p. 5.

[10] *Ibid.*, p. 4.

trends in thinking have done for our mental life what fast food has done to our bodies. If you are sitting there, thinking the same processed thoughts you have been thinking for years, those churned out and spat up by generations long dead, the chances are pretty high that you're out of shape. One need look no further than the major political parties of the Western world to see where this sort of thinking leads.

So what exactly is a conceptual carb? First, as we said, a conceptual carb is not a mental calorie—that is, it isn't a matter of how *much* we think, but *how* we think and *what* we think about that results in our present mental flabbiness. Dr. Atkins teaches us that it is true that you *could* cut your conceptual carbs by thinking less, or not at all, and indeed, this is the path to becoming what John Stuart Mill called "a pig satisfied," a term he used for the politicians he knew. While such persons are not altogether to be envied, there is something to be said for the sausage that can be made of them by the media. But the key to health and to happiness is not to initiate a type of mental diet that we cannot sustain for life. No sooner will you be "satisfied" than you'll find yourself wondering if your daughter has been hiding a tattoo, or some other pressing doubt will assume cerebral residence.

But a conceptual carb? Dr. Atkins says that "mankind is not geared to handle an abundance of refined carbohydrates."[11] What we learn from this, apart from the fact that Atkins was educated before the term "mankind" fell out of favor, and that he thinks the body has gears, is that a certain philosophical anthropology accompanies not only the philosophy of Atkins, but really any broad effort to articulate what makes us better off or worse off, in either mind or body. Later Atkins fills out this view:

> You see, the human body evolved and primitive humans thrived as hunter-gatherers who subsisted primarily on meat, fish, vegetables, fruit, whole grains and seeds and nuts. Candy bars were few and far between. The human body is used to dealing with unrefined foods as they occur in Nature. Consequently, your body's capacity to deal with an excess of processed foods is pretty poor, which is why our twenty-first century way of eating so often gets us into trouble.[12]

---

[11] *Ibid.*, p. 11.

[12] *Ibid.*, p. 48.

The same might be said for our troubles with "conceptual carbs." Translated roughly, we might say that human culture was built upon a sort of education in which thinking for oneself was about as crucial for survival (and for flourishing) as was eating one's own meals. Human culture did not evolve by spoon-feeding already processed and refined ideas to the public. It arose by educating people to think for themselves. The late twentieth century saw the introduction, increasing influence, and finally predominance of forms of communication in which images and information came to be tied together in neat packages—sound bites and photo-ops—that relieve the human mind of having to sort through the information. The image or other packaging of these factoids is what the mind consumes, and the path to forecasted emotional reaction is as direct as is the path from carbohydrate to blood sugar. Thus, we define "conceptual carbohydrates" as any bit of information in which doubt, emotional reaction, and readiness to act are all three presented together, bypassing the normal process of inquiry.

Processed Ideas and Junkthoughts

No source of conceptual carbs is more lethal to the fitness and health of the thinking mind than television. If evolution could have set up for human nature a "perfect mousetrap," it would be television. Humans are like moths to the television flame. Everything in our visual and auditory evolution commands us to pay attention, even to fixate upon the swirling colorful images and pleasing noises emitted from this strange little box. Without ever intending to, we consume the images, experience the emotions, prepare to buy or vote, and never once are we required to think for ourselves. You will derive no more mental benefit from watching Bill O'Reilly or Tim Russert badger their guests than you would derive sustenance from watching them eat. Your brain did not evolve to its present evolutionary condition by consuming the processed thoughts of others. Your natural mental endowment came from much more vigorous activity, solving problems of vital importance to the survival and flourishing of yourself and those you care for. But even the vigorous activity of problem solving is subverted by conceptual carbs.

The marketing and advertising forces have co-opted the relationship between doubt, interest, and action by continually suggesting to you that you actually have problems you need to solve by believing their images and noises just enough to buy and consume their products. Do I have "iron poor blood" or "simple chronic halitosis?" I just don't know. Doubts can be generated in many forms, but the point is that conceptual carbs are processed and complete packages, containing a doubt, an emotional response to it (often fear or sexual desire), and a suggested course of action that resolves the doubt. All of this conspicuously bypasses the normal processes of defining the problem and considering alternative courses of resolution.

Conceptual carbs can be passed on in any way at all, and indeed, they have been a danger to our mental acuity as long as politicians have been making speeches. But just as technology has created the processed foods our bodies are not equipped to digest, technology has saturated our brains with images we are ill equipped to think about. We are no more able to get our minds up off the couch than our bodies, and it is not an accident that television more than any other single innovation is responsible both for our torpid minds and lethargic bodies.

Not by Bread Alone

The key to understanding why the Atkins Diet works on our bodies also may help us unlock the mysteries of mass groupthink. What happens to the ultra-refined processed sugars we pour into our unsuspecting bodies? These excess sugars stimulate a massive insulin release, followed by a crash, and the cycle repeats every time we eat. And, as Atkins says, "for some, the bodily insult of massive insulin release to deal with massive blood-glucose levels has been going on for years, causing the glucose-regulating mechanism in the body to break down, initiating unstable blood sugar and eventually diabetes."[13]

Turning to the problem with our thinking, we might say that the infusion of emotion with our thinking that is evoked by junkthoughts and processed ideas, that is, high-carb concepts, over time renders us incapable of detachment, which is crucial for problem solving. The first victim of junkthought is active imagination; the capacity to stand back from a problem and

---

[13] *Ibid.*, p. 50.

imagine alternatives is indispensable to intelligent problem solving. Over time, those who consume too many conceptual carbs become intellectually diabetic, that is, they become highly ideological, unimaginative, incapable of tolerating intelligent dissent, and governed increasingly by violent emotions in their efforts at problem-solving and decision-making. In other words, they gradually become Republicans and Democrats. It's hard to imagine what would happen to the major political parties in the Western world if everyone suddenly turned off the television and became pragmatists, but it would not bode well for them. The standard ways of disseminating the conceptual carbs are the secret to their success. Just as it is hard to deny that junk food tastes good, it is hard to deny that those who care not for what we think, only for how we spend our money or cast our votes are clever at packaging what they want from us in sights and sounds we can barely resist. It is a problem.

I turned off my television in 1992, having already canceled all newspaper and magazine subscriptions, and going on an Induction program limited to NPR *Morning Edition*, *All Things Considered*, and the *News from Lake Wobegon*. I reached my desired level of diffidence about conceptual carbs and regained the power of independent thinking about two years later. Now I am down to the *News from Lake Wobegon* only, finding that I will be told anything else I really need to know by the news junkies I run across daily. I have recovered my imagination and can watch even a presidential election with detached bemusement. This is as close to happiness as I can imagine in the midst of a decadent, ideological, and violent time. I have witnessed many people I know come to be governed increasingly by fear with little awareness of the reasons for it. I generally recommend that they read John Dewey.

The point to be stressed here is that pragmatism is a sort of diet for our thinking. I believe it has a better capacity to detect the presence and limit the intake of conceptual carbs than any other philosophy, and also to help us avoid their negative consequences. Unfortunately, in the academies often pragmatism becomes a sort of theoretical breakfast of champions, with sugar added, by professors whose interest in practical things is limited to framing a good theory about them—that is, processed pragmatism. Thus, we must distinguish academic pragmatism from pragmatism. We do this in part to prevent a run on the academies by readers of this book, who will certainly be calling up their local colleges and asking to speak to the person teaching pragmatism there. Although I hate to burst anyone's bubble, in my experience, teachers of pragmatic philosophy are not people one can expect automatically to be pragmatic. This would be sort of like expecting Dr. Atkins to be thin. His promise was that *we* would lose weight, and he stated plainly that his "goal is to make *you* become a healthy and happy person and to show *you* how to stay that way."[14] I have a firm suspicion that Dr. Atkins approached this goal in his own life, partly due to his diet, no doubt, even if he carried more than a few extra pounds (as some people suggest). Others bent on discrediting the diet speak as though it were a damning critique of the diet that he may have been somewhat porky when he died (and he succeeded in dying of something other than complications due to being overweight, to his critics' dismay). But no, for a pragmatist, the diet stands or falls on grounds independent of Dr. Atkins's weight. Similarly, please do not measure pragmatism by the lives or happiness of those who profess the philosophy of it in the academies.

The best way to find a real pragmatist is probably to look around you to see who seems above the noisy din carried on by those who are soaring or crashing from consuming the conceptual carbohydrates. These people will not be on television or in magazines or newspapers. Nothing they have to say will fit its time and space constraints. If you think you know such a person, and if he or she seems to know something you don't, try turning off your television for a while, consuming only the news you actually intend to act upon, and only the entertainment that actually improves your imagination and creativity. Don't be surprised if the world begins to look different in a few months.

---

[14] *Ibid.*, p. 7.

2

Nietzsche and the Art of Eating: A Sound Mind in an Atkins Body

WILLIAM IRWIN

With the satirical headline "New Nietzschian Diet Lets You Eat Whatever You Fear Most," *The Onion* lampooned the Atkins Diet and transformed Friedrich Nietzsche's (1844–1900) famous proclamation "God is dead" into the low-carb mantra "Fat is dead" (theonion.com). "Nietzsche," by the way, is commonly mispronounced as "nee-chee." The correct pronunciation is "nee-ch-ya" and rhymes with "pleased ta meetchya" or "come 'n eetchya dinner." All joking aside though, there is a worthwhile connection to note between Atkins and the philosopher who observed, "the abdomen is the reason why man does not easily take himself for a god."[1] Indeed, Nietzsche's unique take on philosophy and life sheds light on Atkins and proper care for the body and the mind.[2]

"How One Becomes What One Is"

Philosophy has a reputation for being impractical, unconcerned with the things that really matter to people and the way they live their lives. Most philosophers don't have anything to say about how one should eat or exercise, or where one should live, but

[1] Friedrich Nietzsche, *Beyond Good and Evil* (New York: Vintage, 1966), p. 89.

[2] See also Shannon Sullivan, Chapter 5, "Transactional Somaesthetics: Nietzsche, Women, and the Transformation of Bodily Experience," in *Living Across and Through Skins: Transactional Bodies, Pragmatism, and Feminism* (Bloomington: Indiana University Press, 2001), pp. 111–132.

Nietzsche does. As he says, "These small things—nutrition, place, climate, recreation . . . are inconceivably more important than everything one has taken to be important so far."[3] Why does Nietzsche think these "small things" are so important? Because "above all men must learn to live."[4] More so than any other modern philosopher Nietzsche was concerned with how philosophy could serve life, how philosophy could be a way of life. Disturbed by most modern philosophers' aversion to everyday life and the irrelevance of philosophy in most people's lives, Nietzsche lamented, "no one may dare fulfill the law of philosophy in himself, no one lives philosophically, with that simple manful constancy which compelled one of the ancients, wherever he was, whatever he was doing, to behave like a stoic if he had once pledged allegiance to the Stoa" (ADHL, pp. 29–30).

For the ancient Stoics philosophy was "the art of living," a view Nietzsche endorses, and to which he adds that the aim of philosophy is to make of one's life a work of art.[5] The subtitle of Nietzsche's final, autobiographical book, *Ecce Homo*, is "How One Becomes What One Is." Nietzsche argues here, as he had throughout his career, that it is not nature or nurture that necessarily makes us who we are. Admittedly, these forces will dominate us if left unchecked—"As though life itself were not a craft which has to be learned from the beginning and continuously practiced without stint if it is not to breed a crawling brood of botchers and babblers" (ADHL, p. 60). But we ourselves have the power over our own lives, to sculpt and shape them, to be masters of them as an author is of the characters in his novel. Alexander Nehamas, a prominent Nietzsche scholar, says, "The unity of the self, which therefore also constitutes its identity, is not something given, but something achieved, not a

---

[3] Friedrich Nietzsche, *Ecce Homo: How One Becomes What One Is*, in *On the Genealogy of Morals* and *Ecce Homo* (New York: Vintage, 1967), "Why I Am So Clever" 10, p. 256. Hereafter cited in the text as EH.

[4] Friedrich Nietzsche, *On the Advantage and Disadvantage of History for Life* (Indianapolis: Hackett, 1980), p. 58. Hereafter cited in the text as ADHL.

[5] See Tom Morris, *The Stoic Art of Living* (Chicago: Open Court, 2004) and Alexander Nehamas, *Nietzsche: Life as Literature* (Cambridge: Harvard University Press, 1985), hereafter page numbers given parenthetically in the text.

beginning but a goal" (p. 182). As Nietzsche says, "we want to be the poets of our life—first of all in the smallest, most everyday matters."[6] And if philosophy is the art of living, in which we attend to the "the smallest, most everyday matters," this must surely include the art of eating. As Nehamas says, "the ideal case . . . is . . . to fit all this into a coherent whole and to want to be everything that one is; it is to give style to one's character; to be, we might say, becoming" (p. 191).

Hunger: The Body in Mind

Woody Allen once quipped, "If there's a mind-body problem, which one is it better to have?" That's an easy one for Nietzsche. It's better to have a body. As he says, "I am body entirely . . . and soul is only a word for something in the body."[7] We don't have to accept Nietzsche's position to take his point. The metaphysics of how the connection between the mind and body works, the so-called mind-body problem, is of *theoretical* interest. But *that* the connection works is a fact, and the mechanics of *how* the connection works is of *practical* interest. It is not a subject merely for intellectual consideration. We don't want to know how the mind and body interact simply to add to the storehouse of knowledge. We want to know because it can make a difference in how we live. As Nietzsche says, "I am much more interested in a question on which the 'salvation of humanity' depends far more than on any theologians' curio: the question of *nutrition* . . . 'how do *you* among all people have to eat to attain your maximum strength, of *virtu* in the Renaissance style, of moraline-free virtue?'"(EH 1, p. 237). To make of your life a work of art it is not necessary to understand the metaphysics of the mind-body problem or to answer such theological conundrums as "How many angels can dance on the head of a pin?" For Nietzsche's taste, philosophy has become too concerned with such abstract matters of no consequence to "how one becomes what one is." It is, however, highly advisable to pay attention to what one eats and how different foods affect

[6] Friedrich Nietzsche, *The Gay Science*, translated by Walter Kaufmann (New York: Vintage, 1974), p. 299. Hereafter cited in the text as GS.

[7] Friedrich Nietzsche, *Thus Spoke Zarathustra* (New York: Viking Penguin, 1969), Book I, p. 61.

one's functioning. Food is fuel for who we are, and we are at the same time both artists and works of art. We can, for example, imagine Arnold Schwarzenegger following the Atkins Diet in making of himself the work of art he is. Along with driving Hummers and Harleys, consuming red meat and shunning "girly man" food, like angel cake, would fit and further give style to his character.

Many people find that exercise with its endorphin high does as much for their emotional well being as it does for their bodily health. Similarly, many who have long suffered from carbohydrate addiction and blood sugar fluctuation find that Atkins not only lowers their weight and cholesterol but lifts their spirits. Indeed Nietzsche recognized proper nutrition and metabolism as keys to peak mental or spiritual functioning, declaring that the spirit itself is precisely a function of the metabolism. "The tempo of the metabolism is strictly proportionate to the mobility or lameness of the spirit's *feet*; the 'spirit' itself is merely an aspect of this metabolism" (EH 2, p. 240).

Atkins promises that the diet "naturally re-energizes you."[8] People who felt constantly hungry and were frequently moody now find they feel satisfied and on an even keel. Why did they formerly feel so bad? The body rapidly processes carbohydrates into sugar for fuel. A rise in blood sugar trips the switch signaling the pancreas to release insulin, which brings down the level of blood sugar. The problem is that this process does not work perfectly, especially over time. The rapid rise in blood sugar from eating carbs can call for more insulin to be released than is needed. The result is that the blood sugar level goes down too far and we feel hungry again. We're all familiar with this phenomenon in the form of the candy crash and burn. As Atkins describes it, "The result of the process is destabilized blood sugar levels, quite possibly causing fatigue, brain fog, shakiness and headaches" (A, p. 50).

So for the many of us whose insulin and blood sugar feedback loop overreacts to carbs converted to sugar, the high is not worth the low.[9] We do better with fuel that burns more slowly,

---

[8] Robert C. Atkins, *Dr. Atkins' New Diet Revolution* (New York: Avon, 2002), p. 4. Hereafter cited in the text as A.

[9] People have different insulin responses to carbohydrate consumption, with about 25 percent having a very blunted insulin response and about 25 percent

namely fat and protein. After forty-eight hours in lipolysis, burning fat for fuel as in the induction phase of Atkins, "the body suppresses hunger and appetite diminishes" (A, p. 61).

On a personal note, since I was a teenager I suspected something was wrong with my diet, that I would be happier if I ate differently. I felt tired too often and too easily and my mood marched to the beat of my hunger. But interestingly I experienced hunger more in my mind than in my stomach. I needed food not to stop the rumbling in my stomach but to clear the fog in my head. I was periodically restless, irritable, and discontent, and only food would fix it.

A funny thing happened when I began the Atkins Diet: I didn't feel hungry. I was on a diet and for the first time in many years I didn't feel hungry! Sure my stomach would grumble a few hours after a meal, but I felt fine. I didn't need to eat to fix my head, to get a boost to carry on. My blood-sugar level didn't go up and down like a yo-yo. It was stable and in "the zone," as another low-carb diet puts it. I had exercised daily for years without losing weight, but I continued to exercise because it made me feel better emotionally and sharper mentally. Now my diet was doing likewise.[10] Indeed, Atkins claims to quickly and effectively relieve common annoyances such as fatigue, irritability, depression, trouble concentrating, dizziness, and insomnia (A, p. 21). Personally, I slept better and ceased to have heartburn and indigestion, and I suspect I've experienced relief from food allergies. Dr. Atkins would not be surprised; as he says, "For many of you, especially if you're over 40, the most significant revelation of controlled carbohydrate eating is the discovery that some nagging physical ills, from headaches to various aches and pains, have completely vanished" (A, p. 146). Actually, I didn't even care if I lost weight, but I did. And after two years I've maintained a weight of 165 pounds, down from 187 pounds. What's more, my cholesterol went down significantly.

---

having an elevated insulin response. See Barry Sears with Bill Lawren, *Enter the Zone: A Dietary Road Map* (New York: Regan Books, 1995), pp. 30–31. Hereafter cited in the text as Z.

[10] According to Atkins, people may feel tired or weak but only during the first few days of Induction as they adjust (p. 99). For an alternative view see Jennifer Nelson, "It's not PMS: I'm just Hungry," *Chicago Tribune* (12th May, 2004).

It is in an Atkins body that my mind can do its best work. Some starving artists may produce works of genius, but this philosopher knows he has to crack some eggs to make a conceptual omelet. Barry Sears, advocate of the low-carb diet "The Zone," encourages us to conceive of "being well" not as the absence of illness but as functioning at peak efficiency (Z, p. 37). As he puts it, "In the Zone you'll enjoy optimal body function: freedom from hunger, greater energy and physical performance, as well as improved mental focus and productivity" (Z, p. 2). As the Latin has it, "Mens sana in corpore sano"—a sound mind in a sound body. Nietzsche notes that achieving such peak performance, becoming the work of art we are, partly through proper diet, is a delicate balancing act. "The slightest sluggishness of the intestines is entirely sufficient, once it has become a bad habit, to turn a genius into something mediocre . . ." (EH 2, p. 240). Think of Tony Soprano, who consumes every piece of *gabagool*, every girl, and every gangster who gets in his way. Although he is literally a work of art, Tony has lots of *agita*, not to mention free-floating anxiety and fainting spells.

"One Has to Know the Size of One's Stomach"

"It's not supposed to work that way," claim the naysayers. But it did. I felt great and lost weight even though people said I shouldn't. That's one of the things I like best; the diet suits my contrarian nature. Nietzsche emphasizes that we must unify our drives and desires to best create ourselves as works of art. With Atkins my appetite, waistline, and "told ya so" attitude form a perfect symmetry, quite unlike my experience on low-fat diets, which left me at odds with myself, wanting to eat more but believing I shouldn't.

Atkins may not be the best diet for everyone, and that's okay. Nietzsche is not a philosopher everyone finds palatable, and Atkins is a diet not everyone finds suitable to their character. Arnold Schwarzenegger could probably become even more truly who he is by following Atkins, whereas Tony Soprano could not follow Atkins without changing who he is. Nietzsche recognized that characters and bodies differ. His task was to know his body, how it reacted to different food and drink. "One has to know the size of one's stomach" (EH 1, p. 239). In speaking about the consumption of tea, Nietzsche suggests that the individual must find what is best for himself: "Everybody has his own measure, often between the narrowest and most delicate limits" (EH 1, p. 239). And the more unique one's spirit is, Nietzsche believed, the more unique and delicate the balance will be. Regarding nutrition, he says, "depending on the degree to which a spirit is *sui generis* [unique], the limits of what is permitted to him, that is, profitable to him, are narrow, quite narrow" (EH 3, p. 242). So those involved in making the most highly refined works of art of their lives need to be all the more careful of what they consume.

Not everyone is overweight and not everyone reacts badly to carbs, so Atkins is not necessarily for everyone. There is significant difference even among those who need Atkins and find it works well for them. The level of carbohydrates at which one will be stable, no longer losing or gaining weight, one's Critical Carbohydrate Level for Losing (CCLL) in Atkins-speak, varies from person to person (A, p. 85).

In my Nietzschean attempt to produce art, anecdotal evidence was enough to suggest to me that Atkins was worth trying for the sake of the mind, the emotions, and mid-section. The results have, for now, confirmed the evidence. In the long run I could turn out to be wrong in much of what I currently believe to be correct, and so I continue to check, test, and monitor—weight, mood, cholesterol, and so on. I pay close attention to medical reports but, as Nietzsche would advise, I pay even closer attention to my own body.

A Way of Life

Philosophy, as Nietzsche conceived it, is a way of life. Atkins is a way of eating, even a lifestyle, not a temporary diet. People don't seem to "get" that. My doctor asked me how long I planned to stay on the diet. For life, I answered. It's not a crash diet for quick weight loss. Of course this is true of most reputable diets. Consider that "diet" comes from the Latin *diaeta*, meaning a daily routine or way of living. It's a way of eating daily, not a short-term, short-lived hardship plan.

What is natural is not always good, but when what is unnatural fails, trying what is natural is not a bad idea. If we accept as natural that which the conditions of human evolution produced, living well on Atkins means relearning what to eat, learning to give up most of what is unnatural in favor of what is natural. Our bodies evolved to suit a hunter-gatherer lifestyle.[11] If we have any doubt as to whether a food is natural we can simply ask ourselves: Could I get this food "naked with a sharp stick on the African savanna"? (*NeanderThin*, p. 14). We need plenty of exercise and fresh foods. Fruits and vegetables are good, but fat and protein were the prizes most sought by our ancestors. While Nietzsche did not advocate "the natural" or "the good"—he challenged the very concepts—he did declare himself "an opponent of vegetarianism from experience" and reminds us that "a hearty meal is easier to digest than one that is too small" (EH 1, p. 239). Of course one can be both a vegetarian and an Atkins dieter, but it isn't easy. And while one may have ethical reasons for being a vegetarian, "it's natural" cannot be counted among them (*NeanderThin*, p. 195). Indeed, many hunter-gatherer societies, not just the Inuit, could not have made it through a single winter as vegetarians.

Certainly processed grains and sugars have no natural place in our diet. Grains and breads came into the human diet less than ten thousand years ago, and human evolution has not yet adapted to them (*NeanderThin*, p. 192). It probably never will. With Atkins we learn to eat what we evolved to eat. Refined carbohydrates are no more natural than alcohol and can similarly lead to addiction. Our systems may fail to function properly when we eat improperly, and so we need to learn to listen to our bodies, first to find the problem and then to fix it. As Nietzsche says, "There is a parable for each one of us: he must organize the chaos within himself by reflecting on his genuine needs" (ADHL, p. 64). To be in tune with the body, listening to what it tells us, is natural. We need to (re)learn that when we eat properly we will not be hungry again in a short time. We need to learn what full is, rather than stuffed. It's easy to gorge oneself on sweets, not so easy on steak. The body co-operates in sending signals to the mind when we've eaten enough of the right stuff. We simply need to listen.

---

[11] Ray Audette with Troy Gilchrist, *NeanderThin: Eat Like a Caveman to Achieve a Lean, Strong, Healthy Body* (New York: St. Martin's, 1999). Hereafter cited in the text as *NeanderThin*. See also Atkins, pp. 25–26, 29 and *Zone*, pp. 12, 99–101.

Cheating: "And Even Weaknesses Delight the Eye"

As with all diets, there is a temptation to cheat while on Atkins, to "live dangerously," as Nietzsche might say. But for some of us, the body's discomfort is more powerful than the mind's guilt in motivating us to stay on Atkins. Indeed, Dr. Atkins claims that for about half his patients the most compelling reason they report for staying on the diet is not the weight loss (which they do experience) but that they "feel noticeably worse if they stop the program" (A, p. 20). Personally, when I go off the diet, having dessert at a restaurant for example, I don't feel right. The next morning I have a headache and, more importantly, a return to the old kind of hunger—I'm surly and looking for food like a partier with a hangover looking for the hair of the dog that bit him. The sugar-bomb of carbs throws off my equilibrium. As Dr. Atkins says, "Many of my patients tell me that after not eating junk food for months while doing Atkins, the distress they experience when they do eat it has cured them of these urges once and for all" (A, p. 220). Yet, unlike the alcoholic or addict who cannot occasionally cheat without addiction returning full blown, many people can cheat on Atkins without going into a tailspin.[12] However we choose to handle it, there is much to learn from the pain and discomfort of an Atkins-cheating hangover. As Nietzsche sees it, not only can we learn much from pain, but we can make positive use of our weaknesses, sculpting them into the work of art we make of ourselves. As he says, "*One thing is needful.*—To 'give style' to one's character—a great and rare art. It is practiced by all those who survey all the strengths and weaknesses of their nature and then fit them into an artistic plan until everyone of them appears as art and reason and even weaknesses delight the eye" (GS, p. 290).

---

[12] See *Dr. Atkins' New Diet Revolution*, Chapter 26, "Food Intolerances: Why We Each Require a Unique Diet," pp. 338–343. Atkins observes that many of us become addicted to the foods our bodies can least tolerate. Such foods make us feel better for the short run but then make us feel far worse, much as with the alcoholic in his addiction to alcohol. Could this be why Nietzsche advises against consuming alcohol? "Alcohol is bad for me: a single glass of wine or beer in one day is quite sufficient to turn my life into a vale of misery" (EH 1, pp. 238).

Would Dr. Nietzsche Prescribe Atkins?

Nietzsche criticized most previous philosophy for its absolutes in the form of "Thou Shall" and "Thou Shall Not," and he strenuously avoided absolutes in his own philosophy. So clearly the philosopher would not advocate the Atkins Diet for everyone. More importantly, though, he certainly would not oppose it. Indeed given his penchant for opposing traditional ways of seeing and doing things, Nietzsche would have found much to praise in the Atkins ethos.

In closing, while you're feeling good about the work of art you're becoming on Atkins, be mindful of Nietzsche's special concern for self-knowledge. How well do you know yourself? How carefully are you listening to your body? As Nietzsche despairs, "Through the long succession of millennia, man has not known himself physiologically: he does not know himself even today."[13]

---

[13] Friedrich Nietzsche, *The Will to Power* (New York: Vintage Books, 1967), Section 229. Many thanks to Greg Bassham, Eric Bronson, Mark Conard (who got me started with Atkins), Lisa Heldke, Joe Kraus, Megan Lloyd, Kerri Mommer, Cindy Pineo, Aeon Skoble, and Mark Wrathall for helpful feedback on an earlier version of this chapter.

3

How Do You Decide What to Eat? Kantian Reflections on Dieting

DAN DENNIS

Who Are You?

What you choose to eat is of great importance in your life, influencing your health, fitness, how you feel, what you can do, and how long you live. The question is, how will you go about making your decisions, and thus how will you go about deciding what to eat?

The approach that this chapter takes has its roots in the philosophy of Immanuel Kant (1724–1804), commonly regarded as one of the greatest philosophers. Kant thinks that what underlies each individual's decision making is one of the following three ways of being:

1. You can be *fundamentally unfree*: a slave to your upbringing, genes, past experience, external pressures, and so on.
2. You can be *fundamentally random*: *free* to change the sort of person you are, *but* changing without any rhyme or reason.
3. You can be *fundamentally autonomous*: *free* to change the sort of person you are, *and* changing in a nonrandom way, based upon reasoning, investigation, experience, and truth.

Being Fundamentally Unfree

Let's begin by looking at 1, the fundamentally unfree person. Imagine Herbert was brought up by his parents to eat only according to the Atkins Diet. They would feed him three meals a day, breakfast, lunch, and dinner, each time giving him a tasty low-carb, high-protein meal. When he grows up and lives alone, he carries on in the same routine. Perhaps his habits might be modified as a result of external pressures—for example, maybe he starts eating lunch at the staff cafeteria at work because there are no other restaurants nearby, and the cafeteria only serves vegetarian food, or maybe he becomes so short of money he cannot afford to eat so much meat and fish. Still it is just events that are governing Herbert's behavior.

Because Herbert is unfree, if he had been brought up in a different way, for instance, if he had been fed just Italian food, then he would have carried on eating just Italian food. If he had been brought up to just eat junk food, he would have carried on eating junk food. Unlike the autonomous person, Herbert does not stand back and recognize the many alternative sorts of food he could eat, the many different attitudes towards eating he could have, and the impact that his diet might have upon his quality of life, health, and well being; and he does not then seek well-grounded reasons for selecting one rather than another. Rather, he just habitually ploughs on as before. His behavior is governed by his upbringing and past events, so Kant would say that he is essentially unfree.

As Herbert is essentially unfree, he is a slave to events in other areas of his life, too. For example, imagine his parents were thieves with a penchant for fast cars. Herbert will unthinkingly follow in their footsteps, steal whenever he thinks he can get away with it, and spend large sums on fast cars. External pressures may modify his behavior—for example, maybe he is put in prison for a short while and then when he gets out is careful to only steal when there is next to no chance of being caught. However, he does not stand back and consider all the many different ways he could live his life, the different principles he could act on, and the different ways he could treat others; and he does not then seek well-grounded reasons for selecting one rather than another. Rather, he just rolls on as before.

The person who is fundamentally unfree may *to some extent*, at a relatively superficial level, choose rationally between certain options. Thus Herbert may be highly rational in working out how to steal from the bank without getting caught, or how to cook the tastiest food that fits within the Atkins Diet. However, he remains *fundamentally* unfree because he does not seriously question whether or not to continue being a thief or whether to continue following the Atkins Diet. In order to be able to question himself and change himself at the most fundamental level he would need to become free.

Similarly, Herbert may on occasion choose at random between certain options. However, it may simply be his upbringing, experience, genes, and so on that lead him to choose at random on just these occasions, and choose at random between just these specific options. Thus, that he chooses at random on occasion does not indicate he is fundamentally free—he may rather be fundamentally unfree, and merely superficially, occasionally, random.

Being Fundamentally Random

Let's now look at Rita, who is free but fundamentally random.[1] She freely chooses between all the millions of available ways of thinking and of moving, and so is not simply carrying on as she has before. However, because she is choosing at random between all the available options, there is no structure in her thought and movement—only chaos. Her synapses fire at random, her muscles move at random. We can see that she will behave like a maniac, or perhaps just quiver and die. Thus, while this is one of the three options facing you, it is not a very attractive one! Indeed, whilst it's certainly a theoretical possibility, and whilst you could strive to become ever more random, it's questionable whether you could succeed in becoming *purely* random, not least because it's likely that you would die first![2]

Clearly, if someone talks to you, or prepares meals in accordance with the Atkins Diet, then you can know that this person is not fundamentally random, because talking and following a diet are structured activities, and someone who is fundamentally random will not engage in structured activity. Or, to be precise,

---

[1] I'm using "random" in the usual sense here—where paradigm examples of random events are the tossing of a coin or the rolling of dice.

[2] For instance, if you always toss a coin to decide when to cross the road, regardless of the traffic, you will suffer a speedy demise!

it would be so unlikely that a person's muscles moving at random would result in structured activity that when we meet someone engaging in structured activity, we are entitled to assume that person is not acting fundamentally at random—just as when we read a book by an unknown author, we are entitled to assume it was not produced by monkeys typing at random! Thus someone engaging in structured activity must be either fundamentally unfree or autonomous.

Note that being *fundamentally* random in the way just described is different from being on occasion simply *forced* to choose at random between certain options, for this latter is something that regularly happens to all of us. For example, imagine you are trying to drive home as quickly as possible through the countryside, but become lost and come to an unmarked crossroads. Then you are *forced* to choose at random between the roads available. You do not choose to choose at random! And you are not being *fundamentally* random, only choosing at random at a very superficial level, between a few clearly defined options with which you are presented.

Similarly, you may choose at random in a harmless, superficial way. For example, someone on the Atkins Diet might choose at random between two different meat dishes because the pleasant surprise of the random outcome might be enjoyable. Again, however, this is not like being fundamentally random, which involves choosing at random at the deepest possible level, between every possible thought and movement.

Being Autonomous

Kant was the first philosopher to make autonomy central to ethics. (Ethics is the branch of philosophy concerned with the decisions one makes and the way one lives one's life.) Kant lived in Königsberg in Germany from 1724 to 1804. He lived a strict, hardworking single life, but was an entertaining and popular lecturer who gave sparkling dinner parties every evening. Philosophy is unlike science, because in science it makes sense to read recent scientists in preference to scientists from two centuries ago, whereas in philosophy we can learn from great philosophers regardless of when they lived—even if, like the sublime Plato, they lived over two thousand years ago! One infallible rule, to my mind, is that it is better to read a *great* dead philosopher, than a *good* living one! Thus, I heartily recommend reading Kant. Kant can be difficult to read in places, but works that are quite accessible include *The Groundwork for a Metaphysics of Morals*[3] (you can skip the third and final chapter, which many people, myself included, find unclear) and Kant's *Metaphysics of Morals*[4] (read the second half, *The Doctrine of Virtue*, before the first half, because it is more interesting and accessible).

The autonomous person freely chooses between all the ways of thinking and moving that are available to him. In this respect, the autonomous person is unlike the fundamentally unfree person, but like the fundamentally random person. However, the autonomous person is unlike both the unfree and the random person, in that he will question, doubt, reflect, investigate, learn from experience and rigorous honest reasoning, and so on, in order to try to find firm grounds for choosing one way of thinking and acting rather than another. He tends to think that there is something to learn, and some sort of right answer, or best answer, to be found. Hence he will not be a subjectivist or relativist.[5]

Nevertheless, just because you think that there's a right or best answer to be found does not mean you can necessarily find it. Honesty and humility are definitely called for. This is like the situation in science, where there are many questions to which we do not know the answers, though we think that there are answers to be found and we try to find them. If we keep trying to find answers, we may make progress and further deepen our understanding, even though a full and final understanding is so far away that we cannot imagine what it would look like.

---

[3] Immanuel Kant, *Grounding for a Metaphysics of Morals* (Indianapolis: Hackett, 1993). (The German word usually translated as 'Groundwork' can also be rendered 'Grounding' or 'Foundations'.)

[4] Immanuel Kant, *The Metaphysics of Morals* (Cambridge: Cambridge University Press, 1991).

[5] A subjectivist is someone who believes that thinking something right or best is what makes it right or best. A relativist tends to think that what is right or best may vary from culture to culture or person to person. Of course, the autonomous person is sensitive to particular situations and differences, and would not act in the same way when visiting a remote African village as when at a trendy New York party. But he would think that there is still a right or best way to act in each situation (for instance, treating the host with care and respect) and that certain things are wrong whatever the situation (for example, using someone as a mere means or object, or murdering an innocent person).

The precise activity the autonomous person engages in will depend upon what area of life he applies himself to. For example, if he tries to find a new mathematical theory, then he will engage in somewhat different mental and physical activities than if he tries to find a new scientific theory, or tries to compose a great new symphony, or tries to decide what sort of person to be, or tries to decide whether to follow the Atkins Diet. However, there will be something that underlies each activity, namely, his autonomy—his questioning, doubting, thinking, reasoning, searching, striving, reading, experimenting, discussing, and so on—all in pursuit of the right or best answer.

Let's see what this looks like in practice, beginning first with deciding what to eat. If you're autonomous, then you will not *automatically* carry on eating the sorts of things you were brought up to eat, but will rather be free to question and change your diet. You will not merely act on habit or on your desires, but will consider whether to break or change your habits, and whether to ignore or try to change your desires. At the same time, you will not choose at random what to eat or follow mere whim. You won't mindlessly swallow the claims of advertisers, magazines, books, fashion, or even widely respected authorities. Rather, you will think for yourself, investigate the available options, and use your reason, understanding, and experience to decide what to eat, including whether to follow the Atkins Diet. Thus, you will not eliminate carbohydrates from your diet simply on a whim, or because you are not too keen on them, or because a friend suggests that you do so, or because a book on the Atkins Diet recommends it. Instead, you will read widely, weigh the contrasting evidence of friends who have lost weight, consider evidence from the health-care establishment suggesting that the diet may be unhealthy, and do your utmost to build up a rational and rigorous understanding as a basis for making a decision. You may then engage in trial and error to find out how the diet works for you, your body type, your lifestyle, and so on.

The Dan Dennis Diet

As an illustration of autonomy in practice, let me describe how I have come to have the diet that I do. Like many people in Britain, I was brought up to eat toast and cereal for breakfast. Toast is cheap and easy, and cereals are heavily marketed as the sort of thing to get you going in the morning. However, rather than just carrying on in the way I was brought up or responding only to external pressures such as advertising and the opinions of my friends, I experimented with different sorts of breakfast. The first thing I found was that I felt better—in particular, better able to think clearly and concentrate deeply—when I had a cooked breakfast of eggs and bacon. This is the sort of breakfast advocated by the Atkins Diet; however, I did not eat it simply because it was advocated by the Atkins Diet, but because I found it worked for me. When I subsequently found that I feel better yet by having a breakfast of fruit followed after a short break by some easily digestible protein, such as eggs, fish, or tofu, I switched to this two-course breakfast. After reading widely about the body and diet, I concluded that the protein helps my concentration, but that it is better to have the fruit first, because this raises the blood sugar level and gives me energy. Thus, you see that I do not simply follow my upbringing, convention, others' advice, or a diet such as the Atkins Diet set out by others; nor do I choose at random what to eat. Rather, I think for myself, using reason, understanding, investigation, and experience to make a decision for myself. This is, generally speaking, what it is to be autonomous.

For lunch, I have lots of protein because it improves my afternoon concentration, but I feel better still if I first have some healthy carbohydrate to give me energy. I generally have rice and vegetables (perhaps ratatouille or curry) followed after a short break by a good portion of meat. In general, I find it better to have the carbohydrate and protein separately. This is something recommended by Dr. Hay's diet,[6] and I do wonder whether the Atkins Diet is popular not only because eating a high-protein diet helps some people feel better and lose weight, but also because eating protein and carbohydrate together is not

---

[6] See Kathryn Marsden, *The Food Combining Diet* (London: Thorsons, 1993); Jean Joice and Doris Grant, *Food Combining for Health Cookbook: Better Health and Weight Loss with the Hay Diet* (London: Thorsons, 2004). There are other aspects of the Hay diet that I do not follow, but eating carbohydrates and proteins separately, while often inconvenient, does seem to help me think more clearly and creatively, and concentrate better. This is important during the working day, but when relaxing with friends in the evening it does not matter too much, so I don't mind then mixing protein and carbohydrate.

something the body likes—and the Atkins Diet avoids this by largely avoiding carbohydrates! Anyway, in the evening for dinner I do not have much in the way of protein, because, being brain food, it tends to make me too alert to sleep well, so I will perhaps have a salad or soup or something, with a snack shortly before bed, usually toast, which I find helps me sleep. So there it is—the Dan Dennis Diet!

I, of course, do not claim that my diet is the right diet for you to follow. I only say that *if you are autonomous*, then you will question what you currently eat; take into account my thoughts and experience along with other things you read and hear and along with your own investigation, experience, and reasoning; and *decide for yourself* what you will eat.

The Autonomous Life

Let us now turn to the broader question of how to go about living your life. Kant is famous for stating that if you are autonomous—and so think clearly, rationally, and rigorously—your acts will be guided by the categorical imperative. The categorical imperative can be expressed in two different, but nonconflicting, ways:

1. When you select your acts by selecting principles upon which to act, you will select principles that you would choose that all human beings act upon.
2. When you select your acts by selecting ends, you will treat each and every human being "as an end," where this means you will treat each and every human being with care and respect, and will not use any human being as a mere means or an object.

Let's look at each of these in turn, beginning with 1. Kant thinks that *if* you are to do other than just habitually act on the principles you were brought up to act on, *and if* you are to do other than select at random the principles upon which you act, *then* you need some sense of certain principles being right and others wrong, *and* you need a way of working out which are the right ones. Kant shows that you can work out which principles are the right ones by examining the formal properties of what it is for a principle to be right. By this he means that just as the right principles in math are ones that everyone can see to be right and base their calculations upon, the right principles in ethics must be ones that everyone can see to be right, and that everyone can base their actions upon.

For example, if you see the point of view of the victim of a lie, then you will not be able to see the principle "lie when you can gain thereby" as right; and clearly you would not choose to live in a world where everyone is constantly lying. In contrast, you and all others *are* able to see the principle "do not lie" as a right principle, and you and everyone can happily live in a world where everyone bases their actions upon the principle "do not lie." Kant thinks that the autonomous person will follow this line of reasoning, and so be someone who acts on the principle "do not lie."

Kant thinks the autonomous person will apply this same general method to other rules, and as a result will end up acting on rules such as: "don't steal," "don't oppress others," "don't be unfaithful," "don't be gratuitously violent to others," "don't seek to gain through another's loss," and so on.

With regards to 2, Kant thinks that if you treat a human being "as an end," then this means that you invariably treat him with care and respect. You do not treat him as a mere means or as an object, nor do you humiliate him, intentionally harm him, ignore him, or fail to consider his feelings and opinions. You try, as far as possible, to promote his happiness and virtue. Kant thinks that if you make yourself into someone who treats all human beings in these ways, then the way that you treat a given human being on a given occasion will flow naturally from that.

Kant shows that there is no justification for treating just some human beings as ends, but not others. The autonomous person will not do anything without justification if he has a choice, so will not make unjustified, and hence arbitrary, distinctions between human beings. Therefore he will choose to not make such distinctions, and will instead treat each human being similarly, as an end.[7]

---

[7] For instance, if you claim that you should *only* have care and respect for yourself and your family, Kant can ask "Why?" If you reply that is what you have always done, then Kant will point out that this is not a reason for carrying on as before. If you say this is what you desire, then he will ask why you follow your desires. If you say this is what lots of people do, he will say, "So what?" I could go on, but you get the picture.

Of course, your obligations towards your family will be different from those towards strangers, because you stand in a different relationship to them. However, that does not mean that you should not treat a given stranger as an end. It only means that you will in some ways interact differently with her, for instance, you might not spend time, discuss your most intimate problems, or share a house with her. But if, for instance, the stranger was in an accident and needed help, then your care and respect should lead you to help her. Or if the stranger is hungry and undernourished, then your care and respect for her will lead you to offer her food, and if she is a vegetarian, then your care and respect for her and her beliefs will lead you to offer food that she feels comfortable eating. You wouldn't pressure her to eat a meat dish simply because it's easier for you, or because you prefer the Atkins Diet.

To recap, Kant does not tell you how you should act or how you should live your life. Rather he shows that you have a fundamental choice to be either autonomous, or unfree, or random. Thus, if you reject unfreedom and randomness, then you will choose to be autonomous. To be autonomous is to try to learn through investigation, employing rigorous reasoning, understanding, experience, and so on. Kant has faith that if you learn, then just as you will end up thinking that 17 + 18 = 35 and that the earth goes round the sun, so likewise you will end up basing your action and choices upon the categorical imperative. And to act on the categorical imperative is, as we have seen, to both act on principles that you can will every human being act upon and to treat every human being as an end. [8]

But What About . . .

It's important to distinguish between true autonomy and the appearance of autonomy. Thus, the mere *observation* that someone has a certain diet—a junk food diet, an Italian diet, the Atkins Diet—does not tell you anything about why he has that diet or what sort of person he is. For example, imagine Kitty follows the Atkins Diet and is honest. Kitty might have been brought up on the Atkins Diet, and brought up to be honest, so

---

[8] If you are interested in this, you can read more on my website: www.pure-ethics.com.

the fact that she is now on the Atkins Diet and is honest may mean that she is unfree, just like Herbert. However, of course it is also possible that Kitty is autonomous, and that as a result of thinking clearly about the issues has decided to follow the Atkins Diet and be honest.[9] Merely observing that Kitty follows the Atkins Diet and is honest does not enable you to know whether she is unfree or autonomous.

Indeed, she may not know herself. People may think that they are autonomous when they are not. For instance, the egoist may think he has autonomously decided to be an egoist, when in fact all that happened was that he delved within himself until he found what appeared to be a bedrock of selfishness, which he eagerly embraced. However, Kant thinks that *if* he were autonomous, then he would have been willing and able to change all aspects of himself, and he would have thought rigorously about whether to change, which would have concluded in his rejecting egoism and instead becoming someone who treats every human being as an end.[10] Thus, Kant thinks that someone who is an egoist is not autonomous, regardless of what he claims.

If you were able to quiz Kitty about why she acts as she does, then you *might* be able to work out from her replies what underlies her action—thoughtless habit or autonomy. However, whether or not you are able to judge whether someone else is autonomous is not the most important question. Rather, what is ultimately important is *your own* decision regarding whether to be fundamentally unfree, random, or autonomous.

Your Decision . . .

Finally, let's consider the choice you face regarding what sort of person to be. Kant would say that to be someone who is seri-

[9] Thus, becoming autonomous will not necessarily result in you acting substantially differently from the way you were brought up to act, though it is likely to result in at least some changes, and may turn your life upside down (for the better, of course!).

[10] Just as someone who thinks deeply and seriously about arithmetic will no longer think 7 + 8 = 16. Note that some egoists claim everyone is necessarily selfish. For any act you mention, they claim that the person "really" did it from selfish motives. However, they cannot prove what the motives were, so cannot prove whether the motives were selfish rather than unselfish. Therefore they cannot prove that everyone is necessarily selfish, so their claim is empty.

ously reflecting and trying to understand and decide at the fundamental level, you must have a spark of autonomy. The fundamentally unfree person does not have this freedom of choice, and the random person does not deliberate in this way.

The question is whether to strive to be as autonomous as possible. Even if you have a spark of autonomy, much of your life may be unfree, merely conditioned by habit, genes, upbringing, and chance events. But to the extent that you are unfree you just run on habitually, lacking true self-understanding, your life determined by past events. Such a life seems to be without any deeper meaning, significance, beauty, and value. Kant thinks that if you reject this sort of life, then you will strive to be as autonomous as possible. Similarly, to the extent that you choose at random, your acts are meaningless, pointless, mere chaos signifying nothing. Thus if you reject this from your life, then you will strive to be as autonomous as possible.

Deciding to strive to become as autonomous as possible is just the beginning. There remains much work ahead, as you reason and learn, and change yourself and how you act in line with your cogitations. Fortunately, this is the most stimulating, enjoyable, satisfying, and beneficial activity there is.

In conclusion, being autonomous is the precondition for deciding for yourself. To be autonomous is precisely to be free and self-determining. Therefore, when Kant tries to teach people to be autonomous he is trying to set people free, and to give them the tools that they need in order to live the best life that they can. Thus, to return to where we started, whether or not the best life for you involves your following the Atkins Diet is your own responsibility to work out.

Part 2

Fat

(Pre-Atkins)

4

"The Food Nature Intended You to Eat": Low-Carbohydrate Diets and Primitivist Philosophy

CHRISTINE KNIGHT

If you're nostalgic for the simple life, try getting back to nature by following a low-carbohydrate diet for a month or two.[1] Eating like a caveman is—according to the low-carb gurus—"the way human beings are designed to eat."[2] Open any low-carb diet book and you'll see odes to primitive life. According to Dr. Atkins, the fertile Paleolithic landscape was filled with scampering animals and robustly healthy humans—thanks to their low-carb, high-protein diet. Barry Sears, author of *The Zone*, tells us that "in Neo-Paleolithic times both men and women had the bone structures of world-class athletes." And it's the same picture in Michael and Mary Eades's *Protein Power*: humans were vital, disease-free hunter-gatherers, whose physiology only deteriorated when the dreaded carbohydrates were introduced into their diet with the agricultural revolution.[3] For low-carbers, it's these primitive people who are the ideal. Forget celebrities and sports stars: you need to rediscover your "inner caveman"[4] if you want to be slender, strong, and healthy.

---

[1] The quotation in the chapter title is from Robert C. Atkins, *Dr. Atkins' New Diet Revolution* (New York: HarperCollins, 2002), p. 221.

[2] Barry Sears, *The Zone: A Dietary Road Map* (New York: HarperCollins, 1995), p. 99.

[3] See Atkins, *New Diet Revolution*, pp. 23, 26; Sears, *The Zone*, p. 101; Michael R. Eades and Mary Dan Eades, *Protein Power* (New York: Bantam, 1996), p. 402.

[4] This phrase was apparently first used by Lauren Kern in a review of a contemporary dance festival; see "History Repeating," *Houston Press* (7th October,

"Look to the Ancestors": The Noble Savage and the Primitivist Philosophical Tradition

Atkins is by no means the first low-carbohydrate diet in the world, and for philosophers, idealizing cavemen is nothing new either.[5] In fact, Robert Atkins and his fellow low-carbers belong to a philosophical tradition of *primitivism*—loosely defined as nostalgia for an earlier, simpler, and better time—which can be traced back at least to ancient Greece and Rome. The ancient Roman poet Ovid, for instance, describes a pre-agricultural "Golden Age" in which the earth spontaneously and bountifully provides for its inhabitants, who feast on nuts and berries.[6] Ovid's Golden Age is strikingly similar to Atkins's own primitive utopia, thriving with animal and plant life: "Even before the onset of agriculture, the human animal was able, for millions of years, to remain strong and healthy . . . by eating the fish and animals that scampered and swam around him, and the fruits and vegetables and berries that grew nearby."[7]

When low-carb writers like Atkins wax lyrical over "strong and healthy" primitive people, they are unconsciously echoing the Romantic philosophical tradition of the "Noble Savage," popularized by the eighteenth-century French philosopher Jean-Jacques Rousseau.[8] According to Rousseau, humans in their original primitive or "savage" condition inhabited a "state of nature" in which they were not only morally pure and innocent, but physically hardy and robust too. For Rousseau, the process of civilization corrupted not only humanity's morals, but also our physical health: "in following the history of civil society, we

---

1999), at http://www.houstonpress.com/issues/1999-10-07/culture/dance_print.html. It's now used frequently by the online low-carb and body-building communities.

[5] The quotation in the section heading is from Leslie Kenton, *The X Factor Diet* (London: Vermilion, 2002), p. 64. *The X Factor Diet* is a British low-carbohydrate diet.

[6] Ovid, *Metamorphoses*, Book 1, Internet Classics Archive, at http://classics.mit.edu/Ovid/metam.1.first.html. Arthur O. Lovejoy and George Boas also discuss Ovid's depiction of the Golden Age in their classic study of primitivism, *Primitivism and Related Ideas in Antiquity* (Baltimore: Johns Hopkins University Press, 1935), pp. 43–49.

[7] Atkins, *New Diet Revolution*, p. 23.

[8] See Jean-Jacques Rousseau, "A Discourse on the Origin of Inequality" (1755), in *The Social Contract and Discourses* (London: Dent, 1973), pp. 27–113.

shall be telling also that of human sickness," he writes.[9] Like low-carbers today, Rousseau regarded agriculture (along with metallurgy) as humanity's downfall, since it allowed people to produce surplus food and thus build up wealth. From this "flowed the evils of social hierarchy, slavery, patriarchalism, and commerce."[10]

Similarly, according to Atkins and other low-carb diet writers, agriculture has dealt humanity a double blow. Not only are high-carb grain-foods supposedly harmful to human health, but the mass production of grain also sowed the seeds for the commercialization of food production. And it's the food industry that, according to Atkins, is responsible for the glut of poisonous convenience foods, replete with refined flours and trans fats, swelling our supermarket shelves—and our bellies. As Atkins writes, "That packaged refined carbohydrate stuff in the supermarket puts money in somebody's pocket. And it puts garbage into your stomach."[11]

Critical Mass: Challenging Primitivist Philosophy

Critics from many different academic disciplines have raised problems with primitivist philosophy. Most of these critics start from a base of *postcolonial theory*—the branch of contemporary critical thought that deals with racial identity and culture. (I find it helpful to think of postcolonial theory as roughly the equivalent, in racial terms, of feminism. Postcolonialism is an antiracist theory, while feminism is antisexist.) Postcolonial critics are particularly concerned with how colonialism (and subsequent decolonization) has affected the identity and culture of Indigenous and non-Western groups. As part of this concern, postcolonial critics frequently consider the ways in which Westerners—including journalists, artists, and even diet-book writers—have historically represented non-Western peoples, places, and cultures. Many of the techniques the West has

---

[9] *Ibid.*, p. 51.

[10] Peter Coates, *Nature: Western Attitudes Since Ancient Times* (Berkeley: University of California Press, 1998), p. 86.

[11] Atkins, *New Diet Revolution*, p. 221. Atkins doesn't appear to connect the evils of commercialized food production with his own Atkins-brand low-carb convenience foods.

traditionally used to represent its "Other" are overtly racist. Think of stereotyped Asian, African, or Middle Eastern villains in Hollywood movies, for instance. But the idealization of Indigenous people as "Noble Savages" has also been a key pattern in the history of Western culture.

On one level, it's easy to attack primitivist philosophy on purely factual grounds. For example, although the evidence suggests that Paleolithic peoples were indeed physically strong, lean, and free of degenerative disease,[12] as low-carbers claim, their life expectancy was about a quarter that of modern Westerners, and even Atkins admits that the caveman lifestyle was one of "savage deprivation."[13] The benefits of modern civilized life aren't hard to spot: education, the arts, technology, medicine, communications—not to mention the simple comforts of a solid house and a warm bed. For critics of primitivist philosophy, however, the issue is not whether primitivists have got their facts straight. Rather, their first criticism is that, when you look closely, primitivists (like Atkins and other low-carb advocates) don't really talk about primitive life at all, although they might seem to. Instead, primitivists like Dr. Atkins, whether deliberately or unconsciously, say far more about their *own* society than the primitive society they're supposedly describing. As critics like David Spurr, Marianna Torgovnick, and William Adams point out, primitivism is a *self-reflexive* philosophy.[14] An excellent indicator of this is the inconsistencies in the way that low-carb authors like Atkins describe primitive life. At one point in his *New Diet Revolution* Atkins tells us that periods of famine were common for Paleolithic humans. Yet back a few pages he's imagining a primitive utopia bursting with animal and plant life

---

[12] See for instance James H. O'Keefe, Jr, and Loren Cordain, "Cardiovascular Disease Resulting from a Diet and Lifestyle at Odds with Our Paleolithic Genome: How to Become a 21st-Century Hunter-Gatherer," *Mayo Clinic Proceedings* 79 (2004), pp. 101–08.

[13] Atkins, *New Diet Revolution*, p. 23.

[14] See for example David Spurr, *The Rhetoric of Empire: Colonial Discourse in Journalism, Travel Writing, and Imperial Administration* (Durham: Duke University Press, 1993), p. 125. See also Marianna Torgovnick, *Gone Primitive: Savage Intellects, Modern Lives* (Chicago: University of Chicago Press, 1990), pp. 192–93, and *Primitive Passions: Men, Women, and the Quest for Ecstasy* (New York: Knopf, 1997), p. 14; and William Y. Adams, *The Philosophical Roots of Anthropology* (Stanford: CSLI, 1998), p. 89.

of all kinds[15]—without, it seems, considering the need to reconcile these two images. According to critics of primitivist philosophy, this tells us that Atkins isn't really interested in giving his readers an accurate picture of primitive life. Instead, he's using idealized images of an earlier time to criticize his own society: the modern West.

Once Upon a Time: Primitivist Nostalgia

Western philosophers and writers have habitually relied on idealized images of primitive life in order to criticize their own culture.[16] And they have done so with increasing frequency since colonial and imperial expansion brought tales of "primitive" peoples in the New World back to European ears, providing the perfect story-book characters onto which to project all the ideals Europeans saw as lacking in their own society. The classic instance of this phenomenon is Rousseau himself, who freely admits that he constructed the ideal of the Noble Savage in order to criticize the corruption and inequality that he perceived in eighteenth-century European society. "Let us begin then by laying all facts aside," he writes. "The investigations we may enter into, in treating this subject, must not be considered as historical truths, but only as mere conditional and hypothetical reasonings."[17] This tendency towards cultural critique explains why primitivist philosophy so often surfaces in times of "despair and anxiety," such as the primitivist resurgence in modernist art and literature after World War I. As critic Marianna Torgovnick explains, World War I "made people ask the vexed question of how and why the West had taken the wrong path."[18] For critics, primitivist philosophy is one manifestation of our alienation, as Westerners, from the modern—industrial, consumer-capitalist, rationalist—society in which we live, and our desire for a more holistic, natural, even *vital* way of life. Frantz Fanon, one of the

---

[15] Atkins, *New Diet Revolution*, pp. 60, 23.

[16] See for instance Adams, *Philosophical Roots of Anthropology*, p. 78; Alastair Bonnett, *White Identities: Historical and International Perspectives* (Harlow: Prentice Hall, 2000), pp. 81, 88; Spurr, *Rhetoric of Empire*, pp. 125ff.

[17] Rousseau, "A Discourse on the Origin of Inequality," p. 45. This point is also made by Spurr; see *Rhetoric of Empire*, p. 126.

[18] Torgovnick, *Primitive Passions*, p. 10.

founders of what we now call postcolonial thought, explains this in an appropriately nutritional metaphor: "When the whites feel that they have become too mechanized, they turn to the men of color and ask them for a little human sustenance."[19] We can see this yearning when Atkins tells us that people "start to *live* again" when they follow his primitive diet; when he says that "modern life is unnatural"; and when he criticizes food manufacturers for making money from "fake," refined-carb convenience foods.[20]

It would be wrong, I think, despite Torgovnick's mention of World War I, to link the current popularity of low-carbohydrate diets to a post-9/11 cultural anxiety in the Western world. But this is not to say that we cannot see in Atkins, or even in a less extreme low-carb diet such as South Beach, a profound sense of loss in relation to Western culture, and a strong tendency to project those ostensibly lost qualities—such as vitality, authenticity, and simplicity—onto an earlier time. *The South Beach Diet*, in particular, exudes nostalgia for a simpler, slower way of life:

> Once, the carbs we ate were less processed than they are today. More of our bread was baked at home or in local bakeries, not factories, and was made with whole grains, not flour that had been overly processed and stripped of all fibre. Back then, convenience and speedy preparation weren't the highest ideals food aspired to—we were in less of a rush, and home cooking meant starting with raw ingredients. Rice had more of its fibre intact, and had to be cooked slowly. Potatoes weren't sliced and frozen or powdered and bought in a box. Children's after-school snacks weren't limited to what could be microwaved.[21]

Just like Atkins's primitive utopia, *South Beach*'s vision is factually inconsistent, such that it's impossible to pinpoint exactly which era Dr. Agatston might like to recreate. As any low-carb author will tell you, white bread only began to be commonly consumed in the second half of the nineteenth century, with the introduction of high-speed steel roller milling.[22] On the other

---

[19] Frantz Fanon, *Black Skin, White Masks* (New York: Grove, 1967), p. 129. See also Torgovnick, *Gone Primitive*, p. 188; Spurr, *Rhetoric of Empire*, p. 135.

[20] Atkins, *New Diet Revolution*, pp. 11, 191, 25.

[21] Arthur Agatston, *The South Beach Diet* (London: Headline, 2003), p. 73.

[22] See for example Atkins, *New Diet Revolution*, p. 23.

hand, factory-based industrial bread production didn't take over from domestic and local baking until the middle of the twentieth century. To further cloud our attempt to date *South Beach*'s utopian vision, rice consumption in the United States has only taken off in the last ten to twenty years, with the push towards low-fat eating and the growing popularity of Asian-style food. And last but not least, compulsory elementary schooling only gradually became a reality for many American children in the late 1800s, especially for the lower classes. So when exactly were the children Agatston mentions eating those healthy after-school snacks? The 1950s? The 1850s? It's impossible to tell. For the critic of primitivist philosophy, however—as I've mentioned—these factual difficulties aren't the point. Instead, the point is that *South Beach*'s nostalgia is self-reflexive, and says more about what Western society today might *lack*, in Dr. Agatston's eyes, than about any real society of an earlier time. Perhaps, if we consider the above passage, what's lacking in Western society today is a sense of local community. Even the home seems to be missing as a source of nourishment and a symbolic center in our lives. In primitivist philosophy, these are common themes—so much so that critic Marianna Torgovnick describes the desire to "go primitive" as the desire to "go home."[23]

"Better in the Bush": Evolutionary Theory and Modern-Day "Primitives"

All this might be enlightening, but not particularly important, if it weren't for the fact that primitivist philosophy doesn't just encompass early humans who lived in caveman times.[24] Diets like Atkins, The Zone, Protein Power, and "Stone Age" low-carb

---

[23] Torgovnick, *Gone Primitive*, pp. 185–190.

[24] The quotation in the section heading is from Eades and Eades, *Protein Power*, p. 46. "Better in the bush" is the heading for the Eadeses' three-page discussion of Indigenous Australians and diabetes. Despite what the Eadeses imply, diabetes is actually more common amongst Indigenous Australians living in remote areas than in those living elsewhere—see "Summary of Indigenous Health, September 2004" (Australian Indigenous Health*InfoNet*), at http://www.healthinfonet.ecu.edu.au/html/html_keyfacts/keyfacts_summary.htm.

programs such as the Paleo Diet and NeanderThin[25] are just as enamored of so-called primitive people in the contemporary world, such as the Inuit, Indigenous Australians, and Native Americans. For instance, Michael and Mary Eades, the authors of *Protein Power*, wax lyrical over the nutritional habits, longevity, and apparently excellent health of the Inuit:

> Eskimos eat very little carbohydrate, in fact no carbohydrate during the winter, and survive nicely to a ripe old age. Although their traditional diet is composed of a large quantity of protein and an enormous amount of fat, Eskimos suffer very little heart disease, diabetes, obesity (despite the cartoons), high blood pressure, and all the other diseases we associate with a more civilized lifestyle.[26]

The frankly racist idea that "we" are "more civilized" than the Inuit brings us to the second criticism leveled at primitivist philosophy by critics like Marianna Torgovnick and David Spurr: the idealization of modern-day "primitives" such as the Inuit relies on the identification of these contemporary groups with Paleolithic humans. This identification, in turn, is dependent upon evolutionary theory, which entered (and reinforced) the primitivist philosophical tradition as European powers expanded their colonial reach in the East, the Antipodes, and the New World. According to evolutionary theory, while Europeans have adapted, evolved, and developed over the millennia from their primitive state, Indigenous groups (so the logic goes) have stayed the same. From a primitivist evolutionary perspective, Indigenous people are regarded as "remnants" of primitive hunter-gatherer groups from human prehistory. Loren Cordain, the author of *The Paleo Diet*, exemplifies this theory when he describes how the Canadian Inuit "literally were transferred from the Stone Age to the Space Age in a single generation during the 1950s and 1960s."[27]

How the Canadian Inuit "literally" got stuck in the space-time continuum for so many years remains a mystery, but it's as

[25] Loren Cordain, *The Paleo Diet: Lose Weight and Get Healthy by Eating the Food You Were Designed to Eat* (Hoboken: Wiley, 2002); Ray Audette, *NeanderThin: Eat Like a Caveman to Achieve a Lean, Strong, Healthy Body* (New York: St Martin's, 1999).

[26] Eades and Eades, *Protein Power*, p. 9.

[27] Cordain, *The Paleo Diet*, p. 81.

impressive an accomplishment as their recent time travel. Authors like Atkins and the Eadeses reinforce this view of modern Indigenous peoples as "remnants" of Paleolithic hunter-gatherers when they idealize the two groups in virtually identical terms, implicitly identifying them across the millennia. The actual histories (both ancient and modern) of Indigenous peoples are completely obscured by this maneuver, since "primitive" peoples, by definition, are thought to be static and unchanging.[28]

These types of evolutionary argument, and the implications they have for non-Western people, make primitivist philosophy of great concern to postcolonial thinkers. Despite the fact that primitivists sing the praises of so-called savage peoples, their underlying assumptions are highly offensive to contemporary Indigenous groups, in particular. As Marianna Torgovnick points out, the idea that Indigenous groups today are somehow the same as Paleolithic people is a major reason for racist stereotypes of Indigenous people (and people of color) as "childlike" and brutish.[29]

But critics have raised further concerns regarding primitivist philosophy's impact on Indigenous peoples. Earlier in this chapter, I stressed that the factual inaccuracies of primitivist nostalgia aren't really the point, and that critics focus instead on the fact that primitivist philosophy is self-reflexive. In other words, writers and philosophers who idealize the primitive are really commenting on their own culture, rather than primitive culture itself. This *is* indeed the important thing in relation to pseudo-Paleolithic utopias like Atkins's fertile paradise. After all, it's probably unimportant to you or me whether or not Paleolithic humans really had abundant food or were periodically half-starved.[30] But most people would agree that it *does* matter whether a bestseller like *Protein Power* gets its facts right about

---

[28] For ideas in this paragraph, see Adams, *Philosophical Roots of Anthropology*, p. 81; Robert Whelan, *Wild in Woods: The Myth of the Noble Eco-Savage* (London: IEA Environmental Unit, 1999), p. 5; Coates, *Nature*, p. 88; Spurr, *Rhetoric of Empire*, p. 167; Torgovnick, *Gone Primitive*, pp. 186–87.

[29] Torgovnick, *Gone Primitive*, p. 186.

[30] Although it does matter to Paleo nutrition researchers—see for example L. Cordain, J. Miller, and N. Mann, "Scant Evidence of Periodic Starvation among Hunter-Gatherers," *Diabetologia* 42 (1999), pp. 383–84.

Inuit health. The Eadeses' portrayal of Inuit health is correct in some respects: for instance, diabetes is less common amongst Inuit than the general population, in stark contrast to the escalating rates of diabetes amongst other Indigenous groups. But the picture *Protein Power* presents glosses over the glaring health inequalities between today's Inuit people and the non-Inuit population of the countries in which they live. No amount of rhapsodizing about Eskimos' amazing health and diet is going to bring Inuit life expectancy into line with the norms for other Canadians or Scandinavians. Nor will it stop Inuit children from dying at two to three times the rate of other children in the same countries and regions. In fact, it might just make readers think that these problems aren't actually there at all.[31]

Artificially Sweetened History

Like Atkins's "Mr. and Mrs. Caveman,"[32] who remind me more of Fred and Wilma Flintstone than any genuine Stone Age man and woman, *Protein Power*'s Eskimos have little in common with the contemporary Inuit. This is a common pattern in primitivist philosophy, which consistently fails to engage with the reality of the eras and people it idealizes—a major concern for critics.[33] An excellent example of this tendency is found in *The New Glucose Revolution*, a bestselling Australian diet book which—like Atkins and other low-carb diets—advises readers to eat foods with a low glycemic index (or low "GI"): those which have a relatively low impact on blood glucose levels, and are therefore less likely to cause obesity and diabetes. (*The New Glucose Revolution*, unlike strict low-carbohydrate diets, doesn't restrict total carbohydrate intake.) Less rosy-eyed than the Eadeses, at least, Professor Jennie Brand-Miller and her coau-

---

[31] For information regarding the health status of the Inuit, see Peter Bjerregaard *et al.*, "Indigenous Health in the Arctic: an Overview of the Circumpolar Inuit Population," *Scandinavian Journal of Public Health* 32 (2004), pp. 390–95. Particular health problems amongst the Inuit include high rates of infectious diseases—up to ten times the general population in the case of tuberculosis—and tragically high rates of interpersonal violence and youth suicide.

[32] Atkins, *New Diet Revolution*, p. 329.

[33] Spurr, *Rhetoric of Empire*, p. 128; Adams, *Philosophical Roots of Anthropology*, p. 85; Bonnett, *White Identities*, p. 84.

thors tell readers that the particular health problems facing most Indigenous groups today (especially skyrocketing rates of diabetes and obesity) are the result of these groups' particular evolutionary history:

> Because our European ancestors had thousands of years to adapt to a diet with a lot of carbohydrate, they were in a better position to cope with the changes in the GI of foods. That is why people of European descent have a lower prevalence of type 2 diabetes compared with people whose diets have recently changed to include lots of high GI foods. . . . In some groups of native American Indians and populations within the Pacific region, up to one adult in two has diabetes because of the rapid dietary and lifestyle changes they have undergone in the twentieth century.[34]

A postcolonial theorist would point out the racist hierarchy implicit in this narrative: "we" are European, while "they" are not, and the reason "we" are now "in a better position" is that "we" developed agriculture, and hence adapted to high-glycemic index foods, while "they" did not. *The New Glucose Revolution* does at least acknowledge that Indigenous people, such as Native Americans, suffer from diabetes at rates vastly above the norms for Americans of European descent. Just like the Eadeses, however, Brand-Miller and her coauthors are caught up in a primitivist "virtual reality" that hides the political and socioeconomic situation of Indigenous people in today's world. In the passage quoted above, Brand-Miller and her colleagues tell their readers that the prevalence of diabetes among Indigenous groups is the result of "the rapid dietary and lifestyle changes they have undergone in the twentieth century." For anyone with even the barest knowledge of twentieth-century colonial history, this phrase quite literally covers a multitude of sins: the taking of traditional lands; the separation of families; systemic discrimination. *The New Glucose Revolution*'s explanation also obscures the extreme social and economic disadvantage—particularly in relation to food and nutrition—that has resulted from these colonial patterns. The socioeconomic divide between Indigenous and settler populations in countries like

---

[34] Jennie Brand-Miller, Kaye Foster-Powell, and Stephen Colagiuri, *The New Glucose Revolution* (Sydney: Hodder, 2002), pp. 215–16.

Australia and the United States doesn't even rate a mention. Instead, the state of Indigenous health is blamed on evolutionary difference and "lifestyle changes"—politically safer territory. Spurr is just one critic who has pointed out that primitivist philosophy acts as "a deflection from politics," diverting our attention from the power relations that systematically reproduce poverty (and ill health) among non-Western and Indigenous peoples. For Spurr, primitivist philosophy is a mechanism by which Westerners "manage" our collective guilt about the poverty in which so many Indigenous people live.[35] But by giving us safe answers, primitivist philosophy actually helps to maintain the status quo, discouraging us from doing anything about racial inequality.

Back to Nature: The Desire for Our Lost Origins

For critics, one of the most unsettling aspects of primitivist philosophy is the implication that modern-day "primitives" (a.k.a: Indigenous peoples) would be better off if they could somehow extricate themselves from Western culture and "return" to their traditional lifestyle.[36] According to low-carbers like Atkins, it's the Western influence on traditional diets which is destroying the health of people around the globe. Even the French aren't immune: "As their diets become closer to American ones," Atkins tells us, "they are losing some of their health advantage."[37] *The New Glucose Revolution* goes so far as to advise its readers that the best diet for them is one that matches their "cultural and ethnic origins" or "cultural and ethnic heritage."[38] As these examples show, primitivist philosophy is a *preservationist*, rather than *assimilationist*, doctrine. For critics of primitivism, this creates an awkward dilemma, since it's no more acceptable for Western academics to tell Indigenous people that they should assimilate than it is for primitivists to tell Indigenous people that they should go "back to the bush."

[35] Spurr, *Rhetoric of Empire*, pp. 134, 132.

[36] *Ibid.*, p. 139.

[37] Atkins, *New Diet Revolution*, p. 25.

[38] Brand-Miller, Foster-Powell, and Colagiuri, *New Glucose Revolution*, pp. 10, 19, 22.

Surely Native Americans, or Indigenous Australians, or the Inuit, can make up their own minds! But even without taking a particular stance in the preservation versus assimilation debate, critics of primitivist philosophy have raised concerns that the particular brand of preservationism sold with primitivist philosophy is completely unrealistic and naïve. The possibility of a return to some authentic, pure culture, untainted by European influence, is particularly anachronistic and impractical in nations like Australia and the United States, where Indigenous cultures are mingled with those of numerous settler arrivals, and hardly anyone has a "pure" ethnic genealogy. When hybrid identities are the norm, how does anyone retrieve their lost cultural origins? *Which* origins? The low-carb mantra "eat what your ancestors ate" is just as unachievable for Western dieters as it is for Indigenous people.

"Back to the Future": Where to Go from Here?

Do criticisms of primitivist philosophy mean that we shouldn't eat low-carb?[39] Or, for that matter, that we shouldn't buy into any product or activity that draws on idealized images of primitive people and their culture? Personally, I don't think we need to go quite that far. I find it helpful to draw an analogy with another Western movement that—like low-carb—has sung the praises of "primitive" people and asked us all to get back to nature: the New Age movement. Anthropologist Diane Bell has written about the way in which "self-styled New Age Shamans" have appropriated Indigenous peoples' spirituality and sense of connection with the earth.[40] Bell points out:

> There is a bitter irony in turning to indigenous peoples to solve problems of affluent urbanites. In the midst of the wealth of first-world nations, most native peoples endure appalling health problems, underemployment, and grinding poverty. A philosophy of reverence for the earth rings hollow in the reality of toxic waste dumps and nuclear testing on native lands.[41]

If we think about the situation Bell describes, the problem is

[39] The quotation in the section heading is from Kenton, *X Factor Diet*, p. 32.

[40] Diane Bell, "Desperately Seeking Redemption," *Natural History* (March 1997), p. 52.

[41] *Ibid.*, p. 53.

not that Westerners are taking on a "philosophy of reverence for the earth." In itself, respect for the earth is immensely important—but it needs to be coupled with action. The problem, in fact, is toxic waste dumps and nuclear testing on Indigenous lands; the health problems, underemployment, and poverty facing Indigenous people; and *the fact that reverence for the earth means nothing while these are still going on.* I think that we can apply the same message about hypocrisy and willful blindness to the low-carb movement. Eating low-carb is fine, so long as we remember that the very same people whose diet we are modeling are those most affected by the health problems low-carb seeks to cure. Low-carb's odes to primitive life ring hollow in the reality of the obesity and diabetes epidemics facing Indigenous groups, because Dr. Atkins, the Eadeses, and their fellows fail to make this basic connection.[42]

[42] I would like to thank in particular Drs. Heather Kerr and Carlene Wilson for their assistance in preparing this chapter, as well as all those colleagues, friends, and family members who read and commented on my drafts.

5

Brillat-Savarin's Nineteenth-Century Proto-Atkins Diet: A Case Study in Inductive Inference

DANIEL O'CONNELL

I stumbled into the Atkins Diet by accident. Several years ago, I was living in a student house, working on my dissertation, and the two other housemates who lived there at the time were really getting into it. Since we used to cook meals together, it seemed to make sense to begin learning to prepare food that fit with the Atkins Diet, since they were always doing the same, and wouldn't eat food that didn't fit the specifications of the diet. It seemed strange to me at first, but after a time I actually got used to it and dropped a few pounds I had picked up sitting behind a computer much of the day and drinking beers with my friends at night.

A longtime foodie and gastronaut, about a year after doing the Atkins Diet I found myself reading *The Physiology of Taste* (*La Physiologie du goût*) by Jean Anthelme Brillat-Savarin (1755–1826). *The Physiology of Taste* is a famous treatise on all things related to food and eating, first published in France in 1825, a few months before his death.[1] Near the end of this work, Brillat-Savarin includes two meditations entitled "On obesity" and "Prevention and cure of obesity" (XXI and XXII, respectively) in which he describes the condition of being overweight and then proposes possible remedies and cures. Drawn to this

[1] Jean Anthelme Brillat-Savarin, *The Physiology of Taste* (New York: Penguin, 1994). I will be referring to this edition throughout this article. References in roman numerals are to the numbered "Meditations." From now on I will give the citations to this work in the text.

topic, and curious about how such things would be talked about in the nineteenth century, I began with these chapters. His discussion of the food types one ought to avoid in order to lose weight resembles the Atkins Diet to a remarkable degree.[2] For instance, Brillat-Savarin specifically names flour and starch, and especially starch in combination with sugar, as the food groups that contribute in the greatest degree to obesity.

Having read Brillat-Savarin, I asked myself, as someone interested in philosophical reasoning and argumentation, what sort of reasoning he used and what sort of evidence he gave to support his notion that one should stay away from foods containing flour and starch if one wanted to lose weight. What sort of argument would he give for this position, developed in 1825, without the benefit of the subsequent one hundred and fifty years of science and nutrition research? His argument—once one gets past the charming prose, which is not easy—is simply this: having looked into the ways in which animals are fattened, he inferred the fattening properties of flour and starch for animals, and then applied his observations on animals to human beings. Reading this as a teacher of philosophy, however, I asked myself: Exactly what sort of argument is this? And how strong is the argument? Does it hold up under scrutiny?

As it happened, I was at the same time teaching a philosophy class on early modern thought, in which we were reading a work by David Hume, written in 1748, entitled *An Enquiry Concerning Human Understanding*. One passage stood out in my mind, in reference to my question about Brillat-Savarin. In the ninth section of Hume's work, which he calls "Of the Reason of Animals," Hume engages in just this sort of comparison between animals and men. Hume's question is not, of course, what makes them fat or thin; instead, he looks at the degree to which animals might possess reason. It has always been one of my favorite sections in Hume's *Enquiry*, devastating in the brevity and directness of its arguments. I decided to take a look at Brillat-Savarin and David Hume together; to explore in more detail Brillat-Savarin's argument in the twenty-second Meditation of his *Physiology*, and then to turn to Hume for an account of the strengths and weaknesses of this sort of argument. In the

---

[2] This has been noted in the book *Protein Power* by Eades and Eades, although I was not aware of that work at the time.

process, I would also be taking a look at one of the earliest formulated versions of a diet that resembled the Atkins Diet: a low-carbohydrate, high-protein diet.

Brillat-Savarin's "Proto-Atkins" Diet

When Brillat-Savarin talks about dieting, he is very specific; he means a regimen (in the sense mentioned in the last section) involving eating and exercise that we undertake to lose weight, because we are overweight. What he outlines in his Meditations on obesity I am calling, both here and in my title, a "proto-Atkins" diet, because it incorporates key elements of the Atkins Diet itself—specifically the avoidance of what we now call carbohydrates. (Brillat-Savarin calls them "floury foods" and "starchy foods and drinks.")

Brillat-Savarin rates diet the most important element of his regimen, coming before "moderation in sleep" and "exercise on foot or horseback," both of which, he adds realistically, people will not do so readily. He adopts a comical tone, considering his possible audience, and notes that, "to suggest to a fat man that he should get up early is to pierce him to the heart; he will tell you that his constitution would never stand it, and that when he has risen early he is good for nothing for the rest of the day; a woman will complain that it gives her rings under the eyes; they will all agree to sit up late, but insist on staying in bed in the morning; and there goes another resource" (Meditation XXII, Section 107, p. 217). As for exercising on foot, he tells us of its horrors in a melodramatic tone, as described by his patients: "It is terribly tiring, and causes perspiration and the risk of catching cold; dust ruins the stockings, and stones pierce little shoes, until going on becomes impossible. And if, in the course of these various activities, the shadow of a headache appears, or a pimple the size of a pin's head breaks through the skin, the régime is promptly blamed and abandoned, while the doctor frets and fumes" (XXII, Section 107, p. 218). Thus, in the end, given the problems with getting patients to undertake exercise and sleep less, he tells us that, "it still remains to seek another way of attaining the same end" (XXII, Section 107, p. 218).

"Now," he goes on, "there is an infallible method of preventing corpulence from becoming excessive, or of reducing it when it has reached that point. This method, which is based upon the surest precepts of chemistry and physics, consists of a diet appropriate to the desired effect" (XXII, Section 107, 218). So diet, for Brillat-Savarin, is the most important thing when one wants to lose weight and fat. Why rate the diet, rather than exercise, so highly? "Of all medical prescriptions, dieting is the best, because it acts incessantly, day and night, in sleep and in waking; its effect is reinforced with every meal, and it ends up by subjugating every part of the individual's constitution" (XXII, Section 107, p. 218).

So how does his proposed diet work, exactly? His anecdotal style sometimes makes it difficult to be clear on the diet's proscriptions, but he is clear about one thing, above all, which is that one ought to avoid at all costs foods that are floury or starchy. Here are some excerpts from his descriptions, found in Meditation XXII.

"You like soup: let it be clear, *à la julienne*, with green vegetables, cabbage, or roots; but croutons, noodles, and thick soups are forbidden" (XXII, Section 107, p. 219).

"For the first course, you are free to eat anything, with a few exceptions, such as chicken and rice, and the pastry of hot pâtés. Eat well but prudently, so that you do not have to satisfy at a later stage a need which will exist no longer" (XXII, Section 107, p. 219).

"The second course is due to appear, and here you will need all your philosophy. Avoid all things floury, in whatever guise they come; for you are still left with the roast and the salad and the green vegetables. And if you must have something sweet afterwards, choose a chocolate custard, or a jelly made with orange or punch" (XXII, Section 107, p. 219).

For those who can't get enough bread, he recommends at least eating rye bread. He also tells his readers that they ought to "shun beer like the plague" (XXII, Section 108, p. 220). Explaining this comment, he notes that the starch "is no less fattening when it is conveyed in drinks, such as in beer, and in other beverages of the same kind." Not mincing his words, he adds, "The beer-drinking countries are also those where the biggest bellies are found; and certain Parisian families which, in 1817, drank beer for reasons of economy, were rewarded with paunches which they scarcely know what to do with" (XXI, Section 100, pp. 209–210).

These are just anecdotes, however. Most directly, he says in several places, in statements reminiscent of Atkins, that floury and starchy food causes fat to form in us. This, he argues, is plain from the fact that we can also observe it to be the case in animals. He himself says it was in animals, or "outside mankind" that he first "elucidated" his theory that fattening is caused by floury and starchy foods (XXI, Section 99, p. 208). Appealing to common sense, he describes the process of feeding animals starches and flour-based foods when fattening them for slaughter. He also notes that animals that are herbivores do not naturally become fat until they are quite old, become less mobile, and begin to feed or be fed on potatoes. From this, he says, "it may be inferred, as an exact consequence, that a more or less strict abstinence from all floury or starchy foods leads to a diminution of flesh" (XXII, Section 107, p. 218).

So in this proto-Atkins diet, Brillat-Savarin relies not on some complicated scientific discovery (although of course he maintains that his prescriptions are in line with those of physics and chemistry), but instead simply observes what we do when we want to fatten animals, and concludes that, because those sorts of foods cause fat in animals, they are also the cause of fat in us (we being also animals). He also provides anecdotal evidence—too long to recount here—from over five hundred conversations with people who were obese, about what sort of foods they ate habitually and what sort of foods they enjoyed and ate most enthusiastically; their lists included potatoes, breads, floury desserts, and other similarly starchy foods. This evidence serves to support his conclusion, derived from observing the causes of fattening among animals. But what sort of argument is this exactly? And how strong is it, as an argument? A look at Section IX of David Hume's *Enquiry* can help to clarify these questions and perhaps provide some answers.

David Hume and "A Species of Analogy"

As mentioned previously, Section IX of the *Enquiry* makes comparisons similar to Brillat-Savarin's comparisons between animals and humans. Hume begins this section of the *Enquiry* by telling us that he's talking about a specific type of reasoning,

reasoning "concerning matter of fact."[3] This is one of the two species of reasoning Hume has earlier identified; the other is reasoning regarding relations of ideas.

Reasoning about relations of ideas is exemplified in mathematics. For example, when we reason, or prove, the Pythagorean theorem, we are talking about the relations of ideas (specifically our ideas of the square on the hypotenuse to the other two squares on the other sides of the triangle). Or when we can say that $5 \times 3 = 30/2$, again this is reasoning about relations of ideas. These reasonings are intuitively, or demonstratively certain; their truth is not a matter of experience. Furthermore, their denial produces a contradiction. It is otherwise with reasonings concerning matters of fact. These are not demonstratively certain, Hume informs us, nor are they intuitively so: the contrary (or denial) of every matter of fact (every *state of affairs* we might say), is possible, since it does not imply a contradiction. For example, here is a matter of fact: I do not have a twin brother. But, Hume would say, you *could* have had a twin brother. There is nothing in your nature, or who you are, that makes it impossible that you might have had a twin brother. To say "Daniel has a twin brother" is not inherently, obviously false. One has to meet me first, and get to know me well enough to find out that I don't have a twin brother in order to verify the falsity of this statement. In contrast, in Euclidean geometry, it is *impossible* to construct a right triangle such that the squares constructed on the two sides of the triangle should not be equal to the square constructed on the hypotenuse. In other words, the contrary of the Pythagorean theorem—"a-squared plus b-squared is *not* equal to c-squared"—is false. The Pythagorean theorem states a relation of ideas.

Consider another matter of fact of which Hume is fond: the proposition "The sun *will not* rise tomorrow" is just as understandable, and does not imply any more contradiction, than the proposition, "The sun *will* rise tomorrow." Now, we may well know, from long experience, that it is highly unlikely that the sun will not rise tomorrow, but this is an expectation, an expec-

---

[3] David Hume, *An Enquiry Concerning Human Understanding* (Leeds Electronic Texts, 2000) (based upon the Selby-Bigge edition), Section XI, p. 104 (http://etext.leeds.ac.uk/hume/ehu/ehupbsb.htm). References will be to section numbers and page numbers as they exist in this online edition.

tation that arises from our experience. Even with the benefit of modern astronomy and all its discoveries, what Hume says here remains true: there is nothing in the proposition, "The sun will not rise tomorrow," that is inherently contradictory or intuitively false. We only expect it to rise tomorrow because we expect the same effects from the same causes. This sort of reasoning, about matters of fact, Hume elsewhere calls "experimental reasoning" (Section IX, p. 105).

It's important to realize that Hume doesn't mean some sort of laboratory work when he speaks of "experimental reasoning"—although one should, according to him, bring this sort of thinking into the laboratory, since physics and chemistry also deal with matters of fact rather than relations of ideas. The word "experimental" meant something quite different in eighteenth-century English from what it means today. It meant something more like "experiential" or "related to experience." So for Hume, "experimental reasoning" might better be rendered today as "experiential reasoning" or "reasoning about matter of fact." I'll refer to it that way from here on out.

Hume thought that we must use some sort of habitual reasoning when we reason about matters of fact. It is this type of reasoning that guides us in everyday life and in understanding the world around us. Hume describes this sort of movement as being founded on a "species of Analogy" (Section IX, p. 104). This species of analogy, as described, "leads us to expect from any cause the same events, which we have observed to result from similar causes" (Section IX, p. 104). Thus, if I eat a loaf of bread from the Brotzeit Bakery on Fleischer Street one day, and it tastes good, and doesn't do me any harm, then I go back the next day and see the same kind of loaf, with the same color and outward appearance, I buy it with the expectation that the same effects (nourishment, good taste, and so on) will result from my eating this loaf. Similarly, a child once burned on the stove in his mother's kitchen will not make the same mistake twice. When the burner is red-hot, or the flame of the gas is visible, he knows not to touch it. In Hume's words, the child "expect[s] from any cause"—in this case the red-hot burner—"the same events which [he has] observed to result from similar causes" (Section IX, p. 104). One critical point to be made here, however, is that Hume did not see this sort of reasoning as a surefire way to the truth. This sort of reasoning, while it usually serves us fairly well in everyday life, could be mistaken. It is, as philosophers and logicians coming after Hume have also acknowledged, a probable course of reasoning, and not one that leads to certain knowledge.

Reasoning by analogy, which we use in daily life, must also be used in the physical sciences, and in all practical arts and sciences such as medicine and dietetics. After all, without oversimplifying too much, it is fair to say the things that such sciences address (such as stars, planets, and even particles of matter too small to see) are likewise "matters of fact," or things we find—or can find—around us in the world. This leads to the conclusion that all the conclusions of the exact sciences are at best probable. Hume provides in this same section of his *Enquiry* an example of such thinking applied to biological science, writing that, "The anatomical observations, formed upon one animal, are, by this species of reasoning, extended to all animals; and it is certain, that when the circulation of the blood, for instance, is clearly proved to have place in one creature, as a frog, or fish, it forms a strong presumption, that the same principle has place in all. These analogical observations may be carried farther, even to this science, of which we are now treating" (Section IX, p. 104). Thus, in addition to his example involving circulatory systems, Hume even finds that he is doing that very thing as he is writing this section of his *Enquiry*, that is, making the leap, by analogical reasoning, from characteristics found in animals to characteristics found in humans.

Brillat-Savarin, it would seem, is doing a similar thing in coming up with his proto-Atkins diet. He observes the causes of fat in domestic animals—that is, the techniques that farmers use to fatten an animal. Then, using the principle of "same cause, similar effects," he applies the idea to human beings, proposing that the same things (floury and starchy foods) that cause fatness in animals will cause fatness in humans. He then makes what he calls a deduction, to the idea that those wishing to avoid becoming fat or those who would lose the fat they have already acquired should avoid such foods, or even the same things in liquid forms, such as beer, and should drink wine instead.

What sort of thinking, logically speaking, allows Brillat-Savarin (or Hume, for that matter) to draw these conclusions? Brillat-Savarin speaks of deduction after he has discovered the principle that carbohydrates (or, in his terms, floury and starchy foods) cause fatness. But he also talks about inference. What is deduction here, what is inference, and how do they relate to Hume's "species of Analogy," which leads us to expect similar events from similar causes?

The sort of reasoning that Hume is talking about when he describes a "species of Analogy" in our thinking is what we can call a type of induction, or what is also sometimes called inductive inference. To make an induction, or inductive inference, at its most basic level, is to say that because all observed A's are B, then all A's are B. Here is a common example of inductive inference: if all observed ravens are black, then all ravens are black. As Hume himself notes, however, the more complex the induction gets, the more difficult it is to be certain that such an induction is legitimate (or will lead to a conclusion that is true). Can we, for instance, conclude from the fact that, because the off-shore underwater earthquake in the Indian Ocean caused a tsunami, that all off-shore underwater earthquakes cause tsunamis? This would be false, as the earthquake some time later near the coast of Japan showed. It must be a certain sort of off-shore, underwater earthquake which causes tsunamis, not just any off-shore, underwater earthquake.

A more complex type of inductive inference is represented by the inference by analogy. This states that certain items—like, say, my loaves of bread from the baker—have properties: say, (a) an oblong shape, (b) a brownish-whitish color, (c) a light but solid crust, and (d) an edible and nourishing nature. These properties, Hume would say, I connect to one another in my thinking, through experience. Then, if I come across another thing, which has properties (a), (b), and (c), I conclude that it also has property (d), namely, that it is nourishing when eaten. This is the "species of Analogy" of which Hume is speaking in his *Enquiry*, and it is also the sort of analogical inference Brillat-Savarin uses. He observes that certain types of food (floury and starchy) are used to fatten animals on farms, and concludes from this that, since we are also animals, and therefore presumably have a digestive system that is at least similar in many respects to animals, we are fattened by similar foods. It is this analogical inference that then provides one of the two premises for his deduction, which then forms the basis for his proto-Atkins diet.

The deduction is a further step he makes, based on the analogical inference. A deduction, at least at its most simple, is a form of reasoning from certain premises to another premise different from the two premises already known. According to the *Routledge Encyclopedia of Philosophy Online*, the Greek philosopher Aristotle, in his work the *Prior Analytics*, has the following to say about deduction (*syllogismos*; literally, "reasoning," hence the standard term "syllogism"). This is an argument in which, if propositions *p* and *q* are assumed, something else *r*, different from *p* and *q*, follows necessarily because of the truth of *p* and *q* (*Prior Analytics* 24b18–20, paraphrased).[4] It's just this sort of deduction to which Brillat-Savarin is referring when he writes that "it may be inferred,[5] as an exact consequence, that a more or less strict abstinence from all floury or starchy food leads to a diminution of flesh" (XXII, Section 107, p. 218). He makes his deduction from two premises: (p) floury and starchy foods cause fat to form in humans; (q) more generally, if something causes a certain effect, then to remove that cause is to remove the effect as well, so long as that thing is the total or at least a major cause of the effect. From these two premises, he deduces the conclusion (r) it would lead to the diminution of flesh (that is, loss of weight), if we removed such foods from our diet. This is the part of his argument that is based on deduction.

The Evidence and Arguments of Diets

What have we seen here? Something quite simple, at bottom. By examining the writings of Brillat-Savarin, we have discovered an early diet that resembles, in key respects, the Atkins Diet. Then, by comparison to David Hume and his "species of Analogy," we have been able to see that the argument that underlies this nineteenth-century diet is not founded on any complicated science, but rather an inductive, analogical inference, based on the

---

[4] T.H. Irwin, "Aristotle," in *Routledge Encyclopedia of Philosophy*, edited by E. Craig (London: Routledge, 1998, 2003). Accessed March 26th, 2005, at http://www.rep.routledge.com/article/A022SECT5.

[5] With this word *infer*, Brillat-Savarin is referring not to inductive inference but rather to deductive inference.

observation of the art of fattening of animals. The conclusion of this inference? Starchy and floury foods, "in whatever form they appear," as Brillat-Savarin says, cause the accumulation of fat in human beings.

The inference is, if we listen to what Hume has to say in such matters, valid, because we are expecting, from similar causes, similar "events" or effects. The cause here, or the state of affairs, is the feeding of starchy and floury foods, in the one case, to farm animals, and, in the other case, to human beings. In the first case, Brillat-Savarin observes, this leads to the fattening of the animal. Thus, he infers, in the second case, it will also lead to the fattening of the (human) animal and, indeed, his conversations with people who are overweight confirm that they have predilections for such foods.

I think that we can see something else here, however, that we can apply a bit more broadly, both to the case of the Atkins Diet and to other diets. That is—following Hume—that diets, and the study of dietetics, deal with matters of fact as well. Dietetics is not an abstract science, in which the principles are immediately, intuitively clear, nor can they be demonstrated like the Pythagorean theorem. Dietetics is a discipline that must be worked out by experimental, or experiential, reasoning, by reasoning about matters of fact, by seeing what works, and what does not work, and by observing the world around us.

One hears an increasingly loud cry, in the newspapers and on the radio, about "epidemic" rates of obesity. Far be it from me to guess whether such statistics may be called an epidemic, but it seems clear that many more people are carrying around much more weight than they were in decades past, and medical science tells us that this only increases the risk of things like heart attacks and strokes.

I myself would not mind losing a few pounds, I must say. I would only bear this in mind, before I rush for the next diet book that hits the shelves: To paraphrase Hume at the end of the *Enquiry*, if we were to go into the section of diet books at our local Borders bookstore, what havoc must we make there? If we take in hand any volume from off the shelf, and ask, "Does it contain any experimental (or experiential) reasoning concerning matter of fact?"—that is, does it contain anything actually based upon anyone's real experience of using this diet, and concerning what sort of foods lead one to become fat or thin? If not, let us commit it to the flames. It can contain nothing but sophistry and illusion.[6]

[6] With sincere apologies to David Hume for paraphrasing this last, wonderful sentence of his *Enquiry* in this context. I take hope, however, from the fact that, if David Hume was correct, then there is no afterlife, and so he cannot see what I am doing nor be angry with me for it.

6

Atkins: Who Gets Philosophical Credit? An Imaginary Dialogue

RAYMOND D. BOISVERT

The Setting: A group of gods, bored with the afterlife, suggest reviving the philosophical "salon." During the 1700s, intelligent, genial women would invite prominent thinkers to their homes for serious conversation. These gatherings became important sources for discussing and disseminating ideas. For their revived "salon," the gods assign the role of hostess to Sophie Boulanger. On her mother's side, Sophie is a distant relation of Mme de Staël, famous hostess who actually coined the word "salon." On her father's side, Sophie is related to Lionel Poilâne, one of France's premier twentieth-century bakers. Maternal and paternal elements are mixed in her name. "Sophie" means wisdom, as in philo-"sophy," literally "love of wisdom." Her surname is a straightforward acknowledgment of the craft practiced by her paternal lineage: baker. For her inaugural "salon," Sophie plans to serve the fluffy, light bread for which she earned her nickname, "la brioche." For the subject of discussion, she has chosen "cross-cultural communication."

THE GUESTS:

Jean-Jacques Rousseau, eighteenth-century French philosopher famous for his political writings in favor of democracy, *The Social Contract* and *Discourse on the Origin of Inequality*, and for his condemnation of modern society as corrupt, hypocritical, and inferior to primitive cultures in his *Discourse on the Sciences and Arts.*

Confucius, the most influential Chinese philosopher, whose impact continues to be felt throughout East Asia, particularly in China, Korea, Vietnam, and Japan. He lived from 551 to 479 B.C.E. Social harmony was one of his prime concerns. His "sayings," *The Analects*, provide guidance in how to become exemplary individuals in harmonious communities.

Democritus (460–370 B.C.E.) was the co-founder of scientific atomism in ancient Greece. Of his many writings, only a few fragments survive. Besides being committed to a scientific or materialistic view of things, Democritus's ethics promoted a life guided by general cheerfulness in the face of fate's many surprises. His most prominent Greek follower was Epicurus (341–270 B.C.E.) from whom we get the adjective "epicurean" (devoted to sensual pleasure, especially enjoyment of good food).

The guests had no sooner arrived than an unsolicited visitor, the mischievous divine agent "Eris," appeared. Eris, strife or discord (not to be confused with "Eros," love), has an infamous place in Greek mythology. Miffed at not being invited to a wedding, she dropped a golden apple into the gathering. On it were the words "for the fairest." Three goddesses immediately stepped forth to claim the apple. The male gods, fascinated by a divine catfight yet frightened lest they face the wrath of the two losers, refused to get involved. Even Zeus, chief of the gods, knew better than to get mixed up in this altercation. He whisked the goddesses off to a land where a young (important fact) man was quietly tending his sheep (young man having spent too much time alone with sheep—another important fact). It fell to him—Paris was his name—to choose the fairest. Not about to take chances, the goddesses all offered bribes. Hera, Zeus's wife, promised Paris wealth and power if he awarded her the apple. Athena, patroness of philosophy, promised wisdom and cunning. Aphrodite, goddess of love, made a simpler vow. If he chose her, she would arrange it so that the most beautiful woman alive would share his bed. The young man, thinking neither with his head, nor really with his heart, and probably tired of erotic fantasies in which the sheep were starting to feature prominently, seized upon Aphrodite's offer. Aphrodite got the golden apple, and Paris was able to woo the woman, Helen. Unfortunately,

Helen was married. Her husband, Menelaus, together with his friends in one thousand ships, sought retribution by mounting a military campaign against Troy. For, as it turns out, Paris was the son of Troy's king. Subsequent events, including gory battles, the Trojan Horse, and Helen's return are all related in Homer's Iliad.

Now the same mischievous Eris who caused all that trouble had decided to disrupt Sophie's salon. Using a tried and true technique, she drops another golden apple. This one says "Atkins."

LA BRIOCHE: Look at this, a household name. This guy's had a bigger impact than all of you. *(Picks up the fruit)* Too bad it's not a real apple. I'm in a cooking mood. What's this? Fine print: "Who takes credit?"

ROUSSEAU: Take credit? Why, that apple's for me. Atkins is only popular because he, he . . . well, let's call it "borrowed" all my major ideas.

DEMOCRITUS: Quite illogical, as usual, Rousseau. Let's examine the facts. *Dr.* Atkins is a man of science. I'm a man of science. Atkins believed in cause and effect. Cause and effect can only be discovered via experiment. Hence credit for Atkins goes to whomever fosters the scientific method. He couldn't care less about unempirical, unverifiable political theories like your "social contract" and "general will."

CONFUCIUS: Self-promotion, like sunlight in the desert, is blinding. You Western thinkers, it's all about "me, me, me." A prize finds its way to the deserving, as a water droplet finds its stream.

LA BRIOCHE: Confucius, you could use a dose of Cartesian,[1] or French, clarity. I'm guessing you all want to fight over a fake apple. What about cross-cultural communication? Well, so be it. Fight over the golden apple if you want. Real apples are the ones I love: Golden Delicious,

---

[1] An adjective derived from René Descartes (1596–1650), the philosopher famous for the phrase "I think therefore I am."

McIntosh, Empire, Granny Smith. And, oh, what my Norman grandfather taught me to do with apples: wonderful ciders, pies, apple flan, turnovers, apple cake, not to mention his favorite after-dinner drink, Calvados.

ROUSSEAU: How can you praise that sugar-loaded stuff? It's unnatural. As Atkins says: follow uncorrupted nature. Look at the date of his first book—1972, the good old "greening of America"[2] era. Remember those days: communes, liberation from outdated constraints, rejection of hypocrisy, Earth day, natural foods, authenticity, organic this, organic that. How could Atkins not have been affected? His focus was the natural-processed split. Look at how he criticizes anything artificial: refined sugar, white flour (there go your grandfather's pastries), sodas, and packaged foods. The Green movement, the Hippie movement, the commune movement, the whole back to nature thing, that's all Rousseau, my ideas making a real impact.

LA BRIOCHE: No pastries!! You can't be French. Swiss, isn't it, from Geneva?

ROUSSEAU: Where I'm from is irrelevant. Truth transcends time and place. All I'm saying is that I put the *alter-* in alternative lifestyle. Atkins just echoes me when he claims that, in the past, "nature really did provide for us very well." Read my *Discourse on the Origins of Inequality.* It's all there: an early state of nature populated by free people. Then, agriculture and civilization. Once we became a sedentary, city people, we became kings and queens of codependence. Hypocrisy and superficial standards began to rule. Society became artificial, superficial, and insincere. Who had the nicest clothes, the best house—people were judged by such criteria. We lost our freedom, our authentic natures, and thus our real selves. I admit it, I'm an *essentialist.* There's a real essence to being human and we have covered that over with a false, hypocritical, sham culture. After me, this was called "false consciousness," a distorted self-understanding imposed by the pow-

---

[2] This expression entered popular consciousness in 1970 with Charles A. Reich's bestseller entitled *The Greening of America.*

ers that be, powers that benefit when we seek happiness in what they have to sell.

CONFUCIUS: Who prefers the clump of clay over the piece of finished pottery? Culture is not an enemy of nature. Do not separate everything that belongs together. Nature is the seed, culture the flower. "Return to nature" is a meaningless slogan. We are cultural animals. Cultural practices are natural. No one would need Atkins if people were guided by my sayings, *The Analects.*

DEMOCRITUS: I thought we all (well, not la Brioche) wanted credit for Atkins's success?

CONFUCIUS: The sage clears the path, he does not seek rewards. Following the path means following the rules of propriety, rituals, *li* in my language. Eat only in the company of others, at appointed times, and in appointed ways, thus will detours from the path be avoided. Take the detour, and you are without compass. Americans, for example—there is a people gone astray. They're grazers, not eaters. They are a people without *li.*

DEMOCRITUS: We ancient Greeks got it about right. We loved virtue, rituals, and good government. But we also prized science. Before Plato[3] got it all wrong with his *philosopher* king, I fostered a way of thinking built on scientific fact, enjoyment in life, freedom from superstition, and a critique of unthinking adherence to tradition. Plato hated science because it dealt with the material realm that he wanted to escape. No one seems to have let him in on an iron-clad certainty about human life: escaping the material realm is neither possible nor desirable. Plato dismissed pleasures, especially those associated with food and sex. The body was only a dead weight for him. That's why he never mentions me. I was his real competition. Sadly,

---

[3] Plato (427–347 B.C.E.) is the West's most famous philosopher. One commentator went so far as to declare all Western philosophy "footnotes to Plato." Unlike Democritus, Plato tended to emphasize the nonmaterial side of human life, the "soul" which had access to a realm of pure ideas, what Plato called the "Forms." His most famous book, *The Republic,* suggests that an ideal state would be ruled by a philosopher who understood these Forms.

Plato's texts survived better than mine. Still, I deserve the apple. Rousseau, science-hating descendant of Plato, certainly doesn't. Confucius, rigid follower of tradition, isn't even worth considering.

CONFUCIUS: Public prizes fade, inner peace endures. Who wants credit for a world that needs an Atkins? Romantic individualism (most honorable Rousseau, a big fan), and scientific materialism (that would be you, honorable Democritus) have little to do with cultivated humaneness. Like spices, vegetables, and meats in a well-prepared stew, humans must find the proper recipes for living a life of social concord. The stew is spoiled if one ingredient overly dominates. The *li* alone provide guidance for the right harmonious blending of actions.

DEMOCRITUS: Don't give me that dreamy, airy stuff. You and Rousseau close your eyes to the nitty-gritty of daily life. Let's think of things like curing disease and relieving obesity. That's what will bring happiness. There is only one tool for making this world a better place: science. Thus science is the only road to real happiness. What can the *li* do for people in pain? Nothing. Atkins succeeded because he turned to science. Where would the West be without its scientists? Leucippus and I, inventors of atomic theory, pioneered progress in science. Science gives us universal truths about nature. Confucius deals only with culture, which is artificial and particular. Rousseau repeats the word "nature" over and over again, but his nature is an imaginary, idyllic invention. It's just a Garden of Eden without rules.

CONFUCIUS: Nature cannot guide, it is a jungle without paths. Culture, nature's best product, is our truest guide.

DEMOCRITUS: Only the ignorant deny the nature-culture difference. Unfortunately, ignorance is plentiful. Akins knows that "consensus," as he disparagingly calls popular opinion, will get us nowhere. Confucius, you're not the only misguided one. Take what Rousseau calls the "general will," his label for the decisions of a democratic people. It's just a democratic fantasy. The opinion of the masses often is, heck, most of the time is, dead wrong. Just imagine doing science based on popular opinion!

CONFUCIUS: Stray from the path and all familiar guideposts disappear. Democritus keeps looking for a reality behind appearances. What does he find: atoms and laws of physics. Flesh-and-blood humans disappear. I live in the regular, ordinary world, one where the only human way to be *natural* is to develop *cultural* practices such as good manners, patterned ways of acting, rituals. We need codes by which to organize our lives.

LA BRIOCHE: We would have had a lot less discord had we stuck with the theme "cross-cultural communication." Why don't we break for afternoon tea? My brioches are just coming out of the oven. Try some with homemade jam.

DEMOCRITUS: Sorry, but Dr. Atkins has warned us against dreaded carbs.

CONFUCIUS: I divorced my first wife because she failed to cook rice perfectly. I'm not doing anything that might violate propriety.

ROUSSEAU: How can we break when an enemy of freedom like Confucius has the last word? Follow him and what do you get: robots, creatures always bending to externally imposed rules. Dismissing nature, Confucius gives us packaged behavior. Industrialists, overriding nature, give us packaged foods. Atkins and I are appalled at both. We hate the artificial.

DEMOCRITUS: You know, Rousseau, you sort of make sense there . . .

ROUSSEAU: Don't be too quick to agree with me. You pretend to follow Atkins, but I know you are a carbohydrate freak. I'm the philosopher who complained about the so-called progress of combining technology and agriculture, the move that gave us refined flour and processed sugar.

DEMOCRITUS: What do you mean, a "carbohydrate freak?"

ROUSSEAU: Don't think I'm unaware of how you lived your last days.

DEMOCRITUS: That was long ago. Atkins was several millennia in the future. I was 109 years old; my sister was taking care of me. She wanted to attend a three-day festival. What could I do?

CONFUCIUS: Festival? An important *ritual* I suppose. Your sister was right. Ritual is the lifeblood of civilized life. Take eating. It's social, it's aesthetic. It takes time. You know what Rousseau says about sex in the state of nature: people meet, mate, and move on. Applied to food that same attitude means all "natural" spontaneity, no rules of decorum. That's *inauthentic*. Manners and conventions are authentically humane ways of living together. Democritus isn't much better. Some of his scientific descendants would be happy if we could invent a pill to deal with hunger. They would rejoice in a direct nutrition delivery system that eliminated the time-consuming rituals of eating.

DEMOCRITUS: Don't confuse me with those austere practitioners of self-denial, the folks we call "ascetics." John Stuart Mill[4] is my kind of descendant: he defended science and individual rights. Both stupid conventions and the tyranny of the majority bothered him. I only wish he had given me credit. Ethical naturalism is the way to go: a life built around reason, science, and common sense; one aiming to minimize suffering and encourage happiness. Epicurus, who did give me credit, got it right when he rejected superstition, magic, anything supernatural, especially the gods. They are sources of nothing but personal anxiety and social conflict.

ROUSSEAU: Nobody lets me finish anything. Democritus told his sister to bake bread each morning. He claims to have survived for three days on the odors alone. And now, this carbohydrate addict says he deserves the Atkins apple!

LA BRIOCHE: Bread? Odors? Can't you eggheads enjoy the smells coming from my kitchen? Aren't there any philoso-

---

[4] John Stuart Mill (1806–1873) was both a champion of political liberalism, see his *On Liberty*, and of the scientific method of investigation, developed in his *A System of Logic*.

phers with stomachs and taste buds? Excuse me while I help myself to a warm brioche.

Democritus: What a scientifically unsound way to eat!! Dr. Atkins would not approve. I'm with Rousseau. Live according to nature. Only, as I keep saying, knowledge of nature comes from experimental science, not democratic poll-taking. The people's "general will" *concocts* truths. Science *discovers* them.

Rousseau: Democritus, not only do you fail to heed my famous claim "man is born free, but everywhere he is in chains," but you help forge new chains. Dismissing public opinion is bad enough, but one-sided worship of science destroys freedom. Admit it. You are a "determinist." Anyone completely committed to cause and effect must dismiss free will as an illusion. If every effect has a cause, there can be no real freedom. But look around you at the wonderful things humans can do, if only they *choose* to do them. The human will escapes nature's chains of cause and effect. Your philosophy is okay for the material world, not the human one.

Democritus: Science allows us to predict and control natural events. Prediction and control are prerequisites for genuine planning. What is real freedom but control over future consequences? Who cares about free will? It has never liberated humans from a single disease or invented any technology to relieve hunger and suffering.

Rousseau: People are not docile cows. They are meant to be as free as they were before civilization fenced them in. Atkins got it right when he said we've "been *had*. . . . Had by a mudslide of media propaganda." We've got to recapture the state of nature. Listen to Atkins: "for thousands of years, human beings were in luck." Why? They ate "real" food, not "invented fake food." When Atkins takes his readers back to prehistoric diets, he's talking exactly the same way I did. That is why I deserve the golden apple.

Democritus: "Democracy" means "power belongs to the people." Real power derives from the ability to predict and control. This is real freedom, liberation from ignorance of nature's ways. Science alone can provide it. Democracy by popular opinion is a disaster. Atkins's book is special because it is based on science. Look at his endnotes. He wouldn't bother with such a lengthy list if he thought democratic voting provided the path to truth. "Scientific support for carbohydrate restriction is unequivocal." These are Atkins's own words, "scientific support," not popular opinion. True democracy, really giving people power, has to be elitist. The "general will" is stupid.

Confucius: Philosophers who live in clouds cannot guide emperors. The sage mingles with his grandchildren. You, Rousseau, put your six offspring in an orphanage. You, Democritus, urged people not to have children. If either of you paid attention to family, you'd appreciate the importance of *li.* Children need patterned ways of behaving. Science can't give them these. Rousseau's state-of-nature fantasies think only of adults, and self-centered ones at that.

Democritus: Children are meant to grow up, Confucius. Customs and traditions are part of the infantile, artificial world. The socially constructed world serves no one but those in power: self-interested religious and political leaders. Therefore, to follow ancestral beliefs is to remain a prisoner. The deep, true, real world can only be understood via experimental investigation. Without that, we remain childlike. Maybe that's what Confucius really wants.

Confucius: Tradition does not keep us childlike. It builds a great wall against those who would manipulate. My honorable fellow thinkers believe that abolishing cultural constraints ("guidelines" I would say), will make people free.

Rousseau: Sure. What is freedom but absence of restraints? Like Atkins, I think that when we wean ourselves from the artificial and the contrived, then we become freer and, yes, "natural." As a bonus we also become thinner (Atkins) and happier (me).

Democritus: Not so fast, Rousseau. Tradition is a trap, you're right there. But, don't forget, your democracy is based on blindly following whatever the "general will" of the people decrees. What is this but a recipe for oppression? It creates a new tyranny, that of the majority, and a dim-witted, ignorant majority easily manipulated by demagogues at that.

CONFUCIUS: Like the banks of a stream, customs keep life from wandering aimlessly. You think the *li* are constraints, and their absence means freedom? Take a look at the twenty-first century. Ethnic and even family norms have pretty much disappeared. Is freedom the result? Definitely not! I'll give Atkins credit on this one. He knows how the processed food industry shapes our desires. Without the *li* there is a void. Whenever there is a void, a new force arises to fill it. Atkins identifies the new force: advertising. When advertising rules, people eat the wrong food and too much of it. When people eat too much of the wrong food they get fat. When people are fat, they turn to Atkins. What a mess—all because my *Analects* continue to be ignored. Only the *li* can counteract advertising's power.

LA BRIOCHE: You guys need a serious sugar rush. I'm a little insulted by your refusal of my home-baked goods. Redeem yourselves. Join me in a visit to the neighborhood patisserie. Marcel, the baker, prepares a special Kir royale[5] for me every day at this time. I'll have him serve you his famous profiteroles—cream puff dough filled with ice cream, all drizzled over with rich chocolate syrup. Followed by a glass of Benedictine, that'll mellow you out.

DEMOCRITUS: Chocolate, ice cream, cream puff, thick alcoholic liqueur! Haven't you learned from the science in Atkins? Let's get back to the golden apple and why I deserve it. Confucius's whole world is about artificial constraints. He's out. Rousseau's got that "green" angle going, but Atkins's references to a distant past are just rhetorical fluff. The real meat (if I may use this term) in Atkins is the science. Rousseau would never use terms like "hyperinsulism," "adiposity," and "benign dietary ketosis." Science

---

[5] An aperitif in which some sweet liqueur is added to a glass of champagne.

is the only path to truth. Give the golden apple to the great ancestor of all scientific philosophy—me.

ROUSSEAU: Don't dismiss the "green angle." "Nature is not to be trifled with," says Atkins. What he prescribes is not unlike what was "our diet for millions of years, long before the bizarre dietary habits of the twentieth century were unleashed to plague us." What could be more Rousseau-like than that? This is the pivot on which Atkins's whole analysis turns. The apple belongs to me.

LA BRIOCHE: Well I'm glad that like Zeus in the original "apple of discord" story, I don't have to decide. All I know is that Atkins praises the French and that's good enough for me. As my grandmother used to say: "When you eat, don't worry about your stomach. When you make love, don't worry about your heart. When you do both you won't have to worry about anything." Enjoying my brioche and jam, I've been not worrying about my stomach. I think it's time to close this Salon, send you three home, go upstairs to my husband, and not worry about my heart.

Part 3

Carbohydrates

(Philosophy of Science)

7

Why and When Should We Rely on Scientific Experts? The Atkins Diet as an Alternative Theory

DAVID RAMSAY STEELE

The Atkins Diet has been condemned by the majority of qualified experts—nutritionists, dieticians, and physicians. Although the preponderance of hostile expert opinion has somewhat lessened since the publication, beginning in 2002, of studies which seem to vindicate Atkins,[1] the majority of established authorities still denounce the Atkins Diet and warn sternly against its conjectured dangerous consequences.

The American Cancer Society, American Heart Association, American Dietetic Association, and American Kidney Fund have all issued official statements strongly discouraging the Atkins Diet. And a number of eminent dieticians such as Dean Ornish have vilified all low-carb diets in colorful terms. The venom of the hostility to Atkins can be gauged from the title of one of the leading anti-Atkins books, *Killer Diets.*[2]

At the same time, there are some experts who support the Atkins Diet, or in some cases deliver a mixed verdict, saying that the Atkins Diet is, if not perfect, an improvement on the typical American diet. Advocates of the Atkins Diet sometimes

---

[1] Among many such studies, see Eric C. Westman *et al.*, *American Journal of Medicine* (July 2002); F.F. Samaha *et al.*, *New England Journal of Medicine* (22nd May, 2003); Gary D. Foster *et al.*, *New England Journal of Medicine* (22nd May, 2003); William S. Yancy Jr. *et al.*, *Annals of Internal Medicine* (18th May, 2004).

[2] Laura Muha, *Killer Diets: Are Low-Carb Diets High Risk?* (New York: Chamberlain, 2004).

have letters after their names, including "M.D." and "Ph.D.", and often argue in detail that the reigning dietary doctrine is wrong, citing research and questioning the interpretation of research findings by the dominant anti-Atkins propagandists.

What's the ordinary person, someone with no qualifications in nutritional science, to make of this? Should we automatically trust the experts? And if the experts are divided, should we always go with the majority and turn a deaf ear to dissenting voices?

Sixty years ago, George Orwell became troubled by the fact that he accepted many scientific opinions without knowing the reasoning behind them. Orwell asserted that he, like most non-scientists of above-average education, would not be able to mount very effective arguments against the Earth being flat.[3] He personally did not doubt that the Earth is round, yet he was bothered by the fact that he seemed to be accepting this scientific consensus with the same uncritical trust as the member of a preliterate tribe might accept the pronouncements of its witch-doctor—or the same blind faith as a loyal subject of a totalitarian regime.

When Orwell wrote, most of Europe was dominated by National Socialist Germany and Soviet Russia. In both parts of Europe, the views of the dominant scientific experts were taught in schools, and most experts seemed to accept them.

In the German-dominated area, the official Nazi line prevailed. Not only were some races claimed to be inferior to others, but many theories originated by Jews, such as Einstein's Relativity, were dismissed as pseudoscience.

Meanwhile, in Soviet Russia, a sixth of the world's population were taught that all of genetics was pseudoscience, and that the theories of Stalin's favored biologist, Trofim Lysenko, were correct. Even eminent scientists in Britain and America, if they were politically sympathetic to Communism, defended Lysenko's theories against Mendel's genetics, while all Western biologists not sympathetic to Communism (more than ninety percent of them) favored Mendel, and held that Lysenko was a wretched mountebank.[4] These developments made it clear that

[3] George Orwell, *Collected Works* (London: Secker and Warburg, 1998) Volume XVIII, pp. 521–22.

[4] See David Joravsky, *The Lysenko Affair* (Cambridge, Massachusetts: Harvard University Press, 1970).

there can be a large element of ideological bias in the determination of the expert consensus on various issues.

Dominant Theories and Alternative Theories

The Atkins Diet is an example of an unorthodox doctrine or a dissident school of thought. In this chapter I will call it an "alternative theory." It's a rival system of ideas, in opposition to the ideas held by most experts in the field, as found in college courses, especially textbooks, and in the public opinions of the most eminent qualified people.

Here are a few other examples of alternative theories:

- Advocacy of megadoses of vitamins by Linus Pauling and others;[5]
- Chiropractic;[6]
- Homeopathy (an unorthodox form of medical treatment which recommends minute doses of substances that in larger doses would actually cause the symptoms of the ailment);[7]
- The conspiracy theory of the killing of President Kennedy;[8]
- Creation Science;[9]

---

[5] Ewan Cameron and Linus Pauling, *Cancer and Vitamin C* (Philadelphia: Camino, 1993). The dominant experts are not as dismissive of large doses of vitamins as they were twenty years ago, but they still reject the complete Pauling argument.

[6] Michael Lenarz, *The Chiropractic Way* (New York: Bantam, 2003).

[7] Bill Gray, *Homeopathy: Science or Myth?* (Berkeley: North Atlantic, 2000). Homeopathy, chiropractic, and numerous other unorthodox doctrines are all outlined in The Burton Goldberg Group, *Alternative Medicine: The Definitive Guide* (Tiburon: Future Medicine, 1993).

[8] James H. Fetzer, ed., *Murder in Dealey Plaza: What We Know Now that We Didn't Know Then about the Death of JFK* (Chicago: Catfeet, 2000); Noel Twyman, *Bloody Treason: On Solving History's Greatest Murder Mystery, the Assassination of John F. Kennedy* (Rancho Santa Fe: Laurel, 1997).

[9] Duane Gish, *The Amazing Story of Creation: From Science and the Bible* (Green Forest: Master Books, 1996). A more sophisticated statement of a Creationist position by a number of qualified professionals is William A. Dembski, ed., *Mere Creation: Science, Faith, and Intelligent Design* (Downer's Grove: InterVarsity Press, 1998).

- Noam Chomsky's account of U.S. foreign policy;[10]
- The theory that someone other than Shakespeare wrote the known "works of Shakespeare";[11]
- An alternative reconstruction of Christian history, popularized in Dan Brown's novel, *The Da Vinci Code*, according to which a secret group within the Church is suppressing the fact that descendants of Jesus and his wife Mary Magdalene are alive today.[12]
- The Orgone Therapy of Wilhelm Reich;[13]
- Climatologists who reject the currently fashionable theory of Global Warming;[14]
- Marxist economists, who reject the dominant neoclassical theory of marginal productivity, in favor of the labor theory of value;[15]
- The theory that the U.S. government is concealing a contact with alien spacecraft at Roswell, New Mexico, in 1947, and the related theory that many thousands of people have been abducted by aliens and experimented upon by these aliens in their spaceships.[16]
- Thomas Gold's theory that petroleum is not a fossil fuel, but is part of the primordial substance out of which the

---

[10] Noam Chomsky, *Hegemony or Survival: America's Quest for Global Dominance* (New York: Holt, 2003).

[11] Among leading candidates are Christopher Marlowe (whose early death must have been faked), Francis Bacon, and the Earl of Oxford. For a survey of different views, see John Michell, *Who Wrote Shakespeare?* (New York: Thames and Hudson, 1996).

[12] Michael Baigent, Richard Leigh, and Henry Lincoln, *Holy Blood, Holy Grail* (New York: Dell, 1983 [1982]).

[13] Wilhelm Reich, *The Function of the Orgasm* (New York: Farrar, Straus, and Giroux, 1973).

[14] Patrick J. Michaels and Robert C. Balling, Jr., *The Satanic Gases: Clearing the Air about Global Warming* (Washington, D.C.: Cato Institute, 2000).

[15] Ernest Mandel, *Introduction to Marxist Economic Theory* (New York: Pathfinder, 1974); Michael Charles Howard and J.E. King, *The Political Economy of Marx*, second edition (New York: NYU Press, 1988).

[16] Philip J. Corso, *The Day After Roswell* (New York: Simon and Schuster, 1997); David M. Jacobs, *Secret Life: First-hand Documented Accounts of UFO Abductions* (New York: Simon and Schuster, 1992).

> Earth was formed, and exists at deep levels in superabundant quantities.[17]

These are just a handful of examples plucked at random from thousands of "alternative theories." We could also mention numerous alternative diets, less famous than the Atkins diet and equally out of favor with the dominant dietetic doctrine. Some of these diets, like the Gaylord Hauser, Protein Power, NeanderThin, or Sugar Busters diets, have affinities with Atkins, while some, like the Macrobiotic or Pritikin diets, are virtually the opposite of Atkins.

Dominant Theories Change

The consensus of qualified experts at any one time is very often reversed later. "Crackpot" theories have become scientific orthodoxy. One of many examples is the movement of continents. People have often noticed that, on a map of the world, the coast of South America seems to fit the coast of Africa, as if these were pieces of a jigsaw puzzle. At one time, anyone suggesting that this had some significance, as showing that the continents had broken apart, was ridiculed as a simpleton or a crackpot. Yet today this breaking apart and movement of continents is the established scientific consensus. It's called Plate Tectonics—and you're now an ignoramus or a crackpot if you question it. Another example is the existence of meteorites. At one time, reports of rocks falling from the sky were viewed much as reports of alien abductions are viewed today. Yet all scientists now acknowledge that rocks do indeed fall from the sky.

The reverse has also occurred. The view, maintained in the Bible, that God deliberately and separately created all the various kinds of living things, and did so about six thousand years ago, was widely accepted among biologists until the nineteenth century. In this case what was once scientific orthodoxy has now become heterodox and "crackpot."

It's reasonable to suppose that some of today's important conclusions of established experts are wrong and will in time be dropped. If we were to list all the hundreds of currently

---

[17] Thomas Gold, *The Deep Hot Biosphere: The Myth of Fossil Fuels* (New York: Copernicus, 2001 [1998]).

accepted scientific theories, we could be pretty sure that many of these will be rejected within the next fifty years. This has happened in every fifty-year period over the last few centuries, and no one believes that this process has just now stopped. We expect that many of today's most respected scientific theories (now accepted as "scientific fact") will be discarded by science, though we don't know which ones.

There's a scene in the Woody Allen movie *Sleeper*, where the awakening Sleeper is plied with cigarettes and chocolates by physicians in attendance. Viewers instantly get Allen's point: the reigning opinion among experts has often changed and will probably therefore change again. Expert opinion is fallible and revisable. What they tell you today is dangerous, they will probably tell you tomorrow is life-saving. The fact that most or all experts favor some view certainly does not mean that it is true, or even that it will continue to be the expert consensus for very much longer. So why should we place any reliance on it?

The Problem of Induction

This brings us right up against one of the classic philosophical problems, the problem of Induction.[18] The word "induction" has a number of different meanings. In the Atkins Diet, the beginning phase, where a person first adjusts her eating patterns, is called "Induction." In electronics, there is a process called "induction" which refers to what happens when you move a magnet inside a coil.

We're going to look at a different sense of induction. In philosophy, "induction" refers to a procedure by which we arrive at conclusions that go beyond our experience. For example, having seen thousands of white swans, and none of any other color, can we conclude that all swans are white? Having witnessed a new period of daylight after every night of our lives, can we be confident that the Sun will rise tomorrow? If all the vegetarians we have ever known have been untrustworthy, can we reasonably infer that all vegetarians are untrustworthy?

Questions like these arise in everyday life and they also arise in science. Much of the philosophical discussion of induction

---

[18] See Bertrand Russell, *The Problems of Philosophy* (Oxford: Oxford University Press, 1959 [1912]), pp. 60–69.

has been about induction as a scientific method, but the conclusions apply to all other kinds of knowledge too. Induction has often been described as "going from the particular to the general (or the universal)," as opposed to "going from the general (or the universal) to the particular."

The problem of induction is a matter of logic. Logic is the discipline which examines *what follows from what.* Logic is not concerned with whether statements are true or false, but with what other statements have to be true, *if* a specific statement is true. For instance, if we accept that "all Atkins dieters eat beef" and that "Bill Irwin is an Atkins dieter," it certainly follows that Bill Irwin eats beef. Logic is not interested in whether it's true or false that all Atkins dieters eat beef or that Bill Irwin is an Atkins dieter. Logic is concerned with whether, *if* it's true that all Atkins dieters eat beef, and *if* it's also true that Bill Irwin is an Atkins dieter, it *must follow* that Bill Irwin eats beef.

And it must indeed follow! Logicians agree that if all Atkins dieters eat beef and Bill Irwin is an Atkins dieter, then Bill Irwin eats beef. In the terminology of logic, this is a valid inference: it really does follow. By the way, this particular kind of inference is called a syllogism, and was identified by Aristotle over two thousand years ago. It has been described as going from the general, or the universal (all Atkins dieters eat beef) to the particular (if Bill Irwin is an Atkins dieter, then he eats beef).

The problem of induction arises because science (and everyday reasoning) seems to require going in the reverse direction, from the particular to the universal. Science is concerned to find "laws," universal generalizations which admit of no exception. Of course, there's much more to science than universal laws, yet such laws are crucial to science.

How does science arrive at its universal laws? Traditionally, the answer has been: by observation. But now the problem of induction rears its grinning head. Observation is always of a limited number of cases, not of all cases. How can we get from observation of some cases to conclusions about all cases?

Induction—forming universal conclusions from a limited number of observations—has been discussed by many philosophers, notably Aristotle (fourth century B.C.) and Sextus Empiricus (third century A.D.), but its difficulties were raised most sharply by David Hume in the eighteenth century A.D. Hume pointed out that no amount of observations of one type of thing could ever justify us in concluding that what we observed would be true of all cases of that type of thing. Nor, as Hume also shrewdly pointed out, could it ever justify us in concluding that the general law was even "probably" true.

Hume was convinced that we do derive universal laws from repeated observations, and yet he believed that this was a logically indefensible thing to do. He therefore reluctantly concluded that our habit of coming up with general laws, though unavoidable, was unreasonable. This conclusion was unwelcome to Hume, who had hoped to find a method for discriminating between what he thought would be justified beliefs (science) and what he thought would be unjustified ones (Christianity and other forms of contemptible superstition). Although Hume did go on to describe ways in which this discrimination could be made, he felt himself to be defeated by what he took to be something illogical, and therefore unreasonable, at the heart of the way we all necessarily think.

After Hume, many philosophers wrestled with this problem. Their solutions mostly fall into two categories. One view is that since we cannot logically arrive at universal conclusions from particular observations, the universal conclusions must already be in our minds. We do not find universal laws in nature, but impose them on nature. This approach, developed by Kant, was taken up by philosophers like Fichte, Schelling, and Hegel, known as "idealists."

The alternative and much more common view, traceable in the writings of philosophers like Francis Bacon and John Stuart Mill, is that as we obviously do learn by experience and observation, we must therefore somehow reason by induction, from the particular to the general. Since logic shows this to be impossible, logic must be incomplete. Logic is therefore renamed "deductive logic," and it is supposed that there is some other logic called "inductive logic," which somehow enables us to get from particular observations to universal conclusions. Unfortunately, no such logic has been discovered—or at least, none which commands the general assent of logicians, philosophers, or scientists.[19]

---

[19] From now on, I follow the Popperian or Critical Rationalist view that there is no such thing as inductive logic. For a different approach, which argues that

Popper's Solution to the Problem of Induction

Early in the twentieth century, Karl Popper came up with a new solution to the problem of induction.[20] Popper accepted Hume's conclusion that nothing could ever justify us in going from "the particular to the general," or in other words, from a limited number of observations to a universal law. But he did not accept that there was anything unreasonable about science.

Popper pointed out that while a proposed scientific "law" could never be *proved* or *established* by any number of observed instances (no matter how many Atkins dieters we find who do eat beef, this can never prove that all Atkins dieters, at all times and places, will eat beef), a proposed scientific law could possibly be "disproved" or *falsified* (just one case of an Atkins dieter who does not eat beef proves that it is false that all Atkins dieters eat beef).

This apparently trivial logical point actually has tremendous repercussions. What it means is this: although no amount of observation can show any theory to be true, observation can sometimes show a theory to be false. And this means that, despite the total absence of positive "proof" for any universal theory, not all such theories are equal. It's entirely reasonable to prefer one theory to another, if one theory has not been falsified and another theory has been falsified.

So, where we have to choose between two theories, we should try to think of cases where they contradict one another in what they claim will be observed. We can then try to set up a test, some experiment which will show one theory to be false without showing the other theory to be false. What was striking, and to many quite shocking, about the studies like those cited above in note 1 was that they indicated, not only that the Atkins Diet leads to rapid loss of weight, but also that it causes a significant improvement in blood lipid profiles, superior to the effects of low-fat, low-cholesterol diets. This was a result

---

there is a way to arrive at a logic of induction, in this case on Bayesian lines, see Colin Howson and Peter Urbach, *Scientific Reasoning: The Bayesian Approach*, third edition (Chicago: Open Court, 2005).

[20] Expounded in his *Logic of Scientific Discovery*, which first appeared in German in 1934. A good straightforward account is Popper, *Realism and the Aim of Science* (Totowa: Rowman and Littlefield, 1983), pp. 31–88.

the advocates of a low-fat, low-cholesterol diet had not expected and could not account for—eating more fat and cholesterol (while cutting carbs) lowers your body fat and your blood cholesterol—though it was predicted by Atkins.

The result of Popper's solution is that Hume was quite right to point out that scientific induction is logically indefensible, but quite wrong to conclude that acceptance of a scientific theory entails an unreasonable kind of thinking. The thinking required is entirely reasonable, it conforms to deductive logic, and there is no need to hanker for any other kind of logic.[21]

This Popperian or Critical Rationalist view implies that no theory ever becomes "final." We always have to leave open the possibility that any theory might have to be discarded. But this turns out to be a realistic view of science, for we know that in the history of science some very firmly entrenched scientific theories have been abandoned and replaced by new theories. The most staggeringly successful scientific theory of all time, Newton's theory of space, time, and gravitation, was eventually falsified and replaced by Einstein's theory—though Einstein did not believe his own theory to be true, and predicted that it would in its turn eventually be replaced by a better theory.[22]

The fact that no theory is finally established does not mean that "anything goes." One theory is replaced by another because the new theory survives the collected observations so far, which the old theory could not survive. Unless some of these observations turn out to be mistakes, hoaxes, or hallucinations, a third theory which will replace the second theory must do better than the second theory *and* the first theory. We are not free to go back to the first theory at our whim—if our aim is to get on the track of the truth.

Popper's Critical Rationalism explains how one theory, perhaps false, can be an improvement over another false theory. If a theory has been well tested and has survived, it makes sense to prefer this theory to others. And even though the theory may

---

[21] It's now fashionable to distinguish deduction from induction by the criterion that deduction is certain while induction is probable. However, conclusions stating probabilities can be derived purely deductively from statistical premises: this has no bearing on the problem of induction.

[22] Newton's theory survives as a special case within Einstein's theory: Newton's theory remains a good approximation for a wide range of phenomena.

turn out to be false, it may yet approximate to the truth in many cases. A false theory can be extremely useful, if it is a good approximation to the truth across a certain range of possibilities. Even though we cannot know that the current theory is true, we can know that it appears closer to the truth than its predecessors.

Kuhn's Paradigms

If observations can test theories and show which theories are best, you might think that there would always be complete agreement on which is the best theory. The real situation is much more messy. A good theory often has troubling anomalies, cases where some observations (or conclusions of some other currently accepted theories) seem to go against the theory, even though, taken as a whole, this theory appears to make the best sense of all the observations. Scientists may disagree on just how troubling those anomalies are. They may, in effect, bet on a promising-looking theory being successful, feeling confident that further research will eventually show that the theory does not really conflict with observations.

Inspired by Popper's solution to the problem of induction,[23] Thomas Kuhn made a close study of "scientific revolutions," historical examples where one firmly established theory was overthrown and replaced by a new theory. He found that in many cases, the existing scientists were not converted to belief in the new theories. They went to their graves defending the old theories. New recruits, young scientists, accepted the new theories, which therefore became dominant as the old guard died off.

Kuhn applied the term "paradigm" to the totality of scientific theories, rules, and traditions in operation in a particular discipline at a given time. He claimed that when a great "scientific revolution" occurs, the majority of existing specialists are so wedded to the old paradigm that they cannot fully understand the new theory. Adherents of the old and the new paradigms

---

[23] Although Popper and Kuhn had sharp disagreements and are usually cast as opponents, Kuhn accepted Popper's solution to the induction problem, and Popper broadly accepted Kuhn's account of the history of physics. See Kuhn's comparison of his views with Popper's, and Popper's reply to Kuhn, in Paul A. Schilpp, ed., *The Philosophy of Karl Popper* (La Salle: Open Court, 1974), pp. 798–819, 1144–48.

"talk past each other," seeing things so differently that they do not identify the same strengths and weaknesses in the two rival viewpoints. Young scientists or scientists from other disciplines are usually better situated to switch to the new paradigm and therefore more fully appreciate the merits of the new theory. (It's notable that a high proportion of low-carb advocates, like Atkins and Agatston, are cardiologists, not dieticians, by background.)

First Question: Does It Ever Make Sense to "Trust the Experts"?

How should a non-expert person make up her mind about what the scientific experts are saying? Right off the bat, one precaution we should take is to check up on whether the supposed "experts" really are the appropriate experts. For example, a doctor, an ordinary practicing physician, may be no more of an expert on the science of human diet than you would be if you spent a couple of hours on the Internet. The doctor may just be repeating the fashionable or official line, without drawing upon any special knowledge. Individuals who have been through medical school and come out with an M.D. have often received very little training in the proper ways to conduct research, and a busy family doctor may not have kept up with the latest research by reading current journals of human nutrition.[24] It's also far from clear that the U.S. Department of Agriculture is an appropriate body to be laying down guidelines on what we should eat.

Assuming we are dealing with genuine experts in the relevant field, our first question is: does it ever make sense to rely upon expert opinion when we don't know what the experts know? Why is it any more reasonable for us to accept what astronomers tell us about the phases of the Moon or what the USDA tells us about the optimal diet than it is for the member of a preliterate tribe to accept the witch doctor's recommendation that he kill his child in order to ensure the rebirth of the sun?

---

[24] Medical experts have a notorious history of scaring people with bogus "health risks." The classic account is Alex Comfort, *The Anxiety Makers* (New York: Dell, 1969).

Here the answer depends upon a theory we hold about the way this group of experts arrives at its preferred theories. If we think that they do this by proposing theories and trying hard to falsify them, subsequently preferring the theories which survive such tests, it will make sense for us to accept the theories currently preferred by this group of experts.

This involves a theory of our own, a theory about the way the group of experts operates. This theory of ours can be tested, and might be falsified. For example, if this group of experts is susceptible to pressure from interest groups, or is prone to make ideological statements about "social responsibility," that would be a sign that they are perhaps *not* subjecting their theories to severe tests. Their views might then quite properly be disregarded, just as the views of National Socialist "racial scientists" and Soviet Lysenkoists should have been disregarded (and were disregarded by most scientists and laypeople in non-totalitarian countries).

It's not the holding of strong opinions that puts a question mark over a community of scientists. It doesn't matter much if scientists are "biased," in the sense of firmly believing in a theory and ardently hoping that it will be vindicated. On balance, this kind of intense commitment to a point of view is probably helpful, though it obviously has its dangers. What matters is the possibility that a community of scientists may be more concerned to defend some theory than to subject it to severe tests. There is no guarantee that a professional community of scientists will not become transformed into a cult-like priesthood, their minds closed to views they classify as heresy. The best protection against such a transformation is open debate.

The more politically or ideologically involved a group of experts is, the more what they say should be looked at closely, for possible signs of dogmatism and blindness to problems in their favored theory. The more they depend upon government money, or money from business interests concerned with the area of their research, the more they should be viewed with suspicion, especially if what they say is welcome to the purveyors of current policies. The Department of Agriculture's experts are unlikely to start a campaign against the near-ubiquity of high-fructose corn syrup. Yet this is a matter of degree, and we should not be perfectionist. Scientific communities have always been subject to ideological and political pressures, and just because they are not pure as driven snow does not mean that everything they say is worthless.

So the answer to our first question, the question that troubled Orwell, is: yes, it does make sense to accept what is currently said by scientific experts in a given field. This is not because of any blind faith in science, or any guarantee that their current theories will not be falsified tomorrow. It makes sense for us to accept—provisionally and tentatively—what scientists say for the same reason that it makes sense for them to accept—provisionally and tentatively—the theory which has done better than its rivals at surviving attempts to prove it wrong. This theory may not be true, it is definitely not the final word of some infallible oracle, but it is preferable to any known alternative, and even if it turns out to be wrong, it will very likely be at least approximately true in many circumstances.

As for the tribal witch-doctor, it may not be entirely unreasonable to accept his recommendations too, in the absence of strong indications to the contrary. But this will be a better bet if there is rivalry among competing witch-doctors and free debate between them, and if they are observed to occasionally revise their "theories" in the light of both observation and argument.

Second Question: Does It Ever Make Sense to Go Against the Dominant Experts?

Science is often presented to children as a triumph of obvious truth over obvious falsehood. The merits of the triumphant view are pointed out, but the merits of the defeated view, and the difficulties which seemed to lie in the later triumphant view, are often not mentioned. While this provides a story that is easy to understand, it can be highly misleading. For example, the theory that the earth spins and orbits the sun was rejected by no less a hard-headed enemy of superstition than Francis Bacon, for reasons which seemed to him very persuasive.[25] The great early astronomer Tycho Brahe also refused to swallow the moving earth. Galileo rejected the theory that the Moon causes the

[25] See Peter Urbach, *Francis Bacon's Philosophy of Science* (La Salle: Open Court, 1987), pp. 125–134.

tides, partly because he considered it an astrological theory of occult forces.

Science progresses by debate and disputation. It is typically untidy and often acrimonious. Significant scientific advances are usually highly controversial. Arguments, even bitter quarrels, between different opinions are therefore not alien to science, and we should never seek to rise above them by appealing to "the established facts," meaning the current consensus of scientists' opinions.

What should the ordinary person do about these scientific debates? So far I have been assuming that there is a clear line separating "the ordinary person" from "the expert scientist." In fact, the division is not so clear-cut. Science is a specialized occupation, just as plumbing or crime prevention are specialized occupations. But some non-plumbers may fix their own dripping pipes, and some non-police officers may shoot a rapist or a burglar. Specialization is only a matter of convenience. Scientists, like plumbers and police officers, are doing something for the rest of us, just because each of us can't do everything.

In fact, many contributions to science have been made by unqualified amateurs or people on the fringes of a scientific profession, and there is some evidence that specialized disciplines sealed off from interaction with the general public become hidebound and sterile.[26] There are also valuable contributions by scholars in disciplines other than their own narrow specialty. Kuhn, as we have seen, claimed that major innovations are more likely to be made by outsiders, and many historians of science agree with Kuhn. Experts in specialized disciplines often find that explaining their theories to the general public helps them to develop those very theories, and in some cases, genuine new contributions are made by works aimed at a broad popular audience, a good example being the best-selling books of Richard Dawkins on evolutionary biology.[27]

---

[26] See W.W. Bartley III, *Unfathomed Knowledge, Unmeasured Wealth: On Universities and the Wealth of Nations* (La Salle: Open Court, 1990), pp. 120–142.

[27] Dawkins's concept of the "meme" has now been adopted in several social-science disciplines. It was first propounded in his popular work, *The Selfish Gene* (Oxford: Oxford University Press, 1976).

The progress of science is a social process, involving the interaction of many individuals, and it is an inherently controversial process, advancing by debate, disputation, criticism, and the clash of competing theories. In this process of argumentative exploration, privileging specific groups as uniquely qualified to pronounce on various topics can be harmful. Debate, persuasive advocacy, and confrontation of rival views are not imperfections, but necessary aspects of the growth of knowledge.

When a dominant theory is challenged by an alternative theory, the result may be the revolutionary overthrow of the dominant theory or it may be the continuation of the dominant theory. But it's also possible that the dominant theory becomes modified by its responses to the alternative theory. We see this in the case of the Atkins diet.

Twenty years ago opponents of the Atkins Diet generally claimed that it was not an effective way to lose weight. Few people claim this now: most critics concede that Atkins does work. Defenders of the dominant theory fall back on four assertions: 1. that the Atkins Diet works by cutting calorie intake, and not in the way that Robert Atkins contended; 2. that Atkins's opposition to soda, potato chips, and other refined carbohydrates is correct, but not his strict limitation of unrefined carbohydrates; 3. that there may possibly be long-term injurious effects from a high-protein diet (the most commonly cited of these so far uncorroborated surmises is kidney damage); and 4. that the studies conducted to date have involved small numbers of subjects, and their findings may not be borne out by studies on a bigger scale.

Don't Leave It to the Experts

Should we accept the recommendations of most dietary experts or should we adopt the Atkins Diet or some other alternative diet? I have not tried to answer this question.

What I have claimed is that there is nothing necessarily foolish or wrong-headed about accepting the recommendations of experts in a field about which you know very little. And neither is there anything necessarily foolish or wrong-headed about taking the side of an alternative theory against the established consensus of experts.

Which of these you do in this particular case I leave to you. Read some of the controversy and you will automatically come up with a point of view. This will be tentative and revisable in the light of further information, but so are all theories and all conclusions, expert or non-expert. Jump right into the ongoing debate: what else is your mind for? Human Knowledge is too important to be left to experts.

8
The Nietzsche Diet and Dr. Atkins's Science

REBECCA BAMFORD

All prejudices come from the intestines.

—FRIEDRICH NIETZSCHE, *Ecce Homo*

Atkins devotees know full well that by advocating a low-carbohydrate, high-protein diet, they are flying in the face of popular thinking and official advice.

Most of us have heard, many times over, that we should follow a low-fat, high-carbohydrate diet in order to lose or maintain weight and to live in a healthy manner. This way of eating has been supported by governments, on the basis of scientific evidence which supports the hypothesis that low-fat, high-carbohydrate eating is healthy, and by certain sectors of industry, which have an obvious vested interest in promoting nutritional advice that encourages the consumption of processed foodstuffs. Similar to sugary foods, commercially produced complex carbohydrates are often highly processed.

In his *New Diet Revolution*, Dr. Atkins offers an alternative to this way of eating, a diet based on the idea that highly processed and refined foods, which he believes to have a detrimental effect upon human metabolism, are in fact demonstrably unhealthy.[1] But Dr. Atkins also offers something else.

Although he bases his nutritional advice on scientific evidence, he repeatedly encourages us not simply to accept what

---

[1] Robert C. Atkins, *Dr. Atkins' New Diet Revolution* (London: Vermilion, 1999). All page references are given in parentheses in the text.

he says, but instead to think about the issue of diet and nutrition for ourselves. Rather than expecting us to follow his diet plan without question, he invites us to evaluate its efficacy for our individual needs, and on this basis, to interpret the basic principles contained in *New Diet Revolution*. In this chapter I'm going to look at the importance Dr. Atkins places on individual analysis and interpretation for successful weight control, and for broader cultural awareness of optimal nutrition. The priority that Atkins gives to interpretation in many ways reflects Friedrich Nietzsche's concern to restore a previously decadent, nihilistic culture to health, by encouraging individual interpretation in preference to dogmatic reliance upon science as truth, and truth seen as divine. From the standpoint of his cultural concerns, Nietzsche offers us a critique of science and truth that, while not anti-science, takes seriously the principle that we should think for ourselves and create our own values, rather than simply following long-held rules blindly and unquestioningly.

Nietzsche's Question of Nutriment

It might seem odd to draw together a nineteenth-century philosopher, and a (mostly) twentieth-century diet "guru." After all, Nietzsche is not especially well known for his nutritional advice, and Dr. Atkins was no philosopher.

This is not to say that Nietzsche was unconcerned with the issues of diet and nutrition. In poor physical health for most of his life, Nietzsche was, until his mental collapse in 1889, searching for a lifestyle that would free him from the tremendous headaches, pain, and sickness that afflicted him.[2] For a large part of his adult life, he wandered in the south of France, Switzerland, and Italy, hoping to find a climate and a way of living that would benefit him. In *Ecce Homo*, his final published book, Nietzsche comments that he regrets hearing what he calls the "question of nutriment"—roughly, the question of how best to nourish oneself so as to attain a maximum of strength—so late in life.[3] By "strength," Nietzsche means rather more than

[2] See R.J. Hollingdale, *Nietzsche: The Man and His Philosophy* (London: Routledge, 1965).

[3] Friedrich Nietzsche, *Ecce Homo* (Harmondsworth: Penguin, 1979), II, §1. Throughout, I use the standard abbreviation *EH* for Nietzsche's *Ecce Homo*.

simply physical vigor, as we'll see shortly. But physical strength and vitality, attained through nutriment, are certainly important to him.

Some of Nietzsche's specific views on diet and nutrition, as expressed in *Ecce Homo* (II, §1), would not have offended the principles of the Atkins Diet. Describing himself as an opponent of vegetarianism "from experience," Nietzsche objects to a number of other specific dietary habits on health grounds. He rejects the notion of unnecessary eating between meals, the drinking of coffee (as it "makes gloomy"), and encourages abstention from alcohol—although he notes, amusingly, that strong doses of alcohol almost turn him into a sailor! He directly encourages drinking plenty of water, as Atkins does—although where Atkins encourages us repeatedly to eat as much as we want if we're hungry, Nietzsche points out that a big meal is much harder to digest than a small one. Nietzsche also recommends drinking tea, but only strong tea, and only in the morning, believing that tea is detrimental if drunk, too weak, throughout the day.

Interestingly, Nietzsche's views on nutriment include place and climate, as well as diet. He maintains that no one—including himself—is free to live anywhere, because climate influences human metabolism (a claim that is now borne out by the acceptance of Seasonal Affective Disorder as a medical condition). This view also reflects to some extent the difference between the working culture of the nineteenth and twentieth centuries: unlike Nietzsche, Atkins simply cannot afford to factor place and climate into his nutritional recommendations. Indeed, the burgeoning range of Atkins convenience foods allows Atkins dieters to cater to this aspect of contemporary culture with increasing ease—something with which I doubt Nietzsche would have been in agreement. Nietzsche also claims that the tempo of the metabolism stands in an exact relationship to the relative mobility, or sluggishness, of the feet of the human spirit, which itself is a part of metabolism.[4] In this respect, too,

---

The numbers following all title abbreviations refer to section and paragraph numbers, which are the same across editions.

[4] Some philosophers, such as Descartes, are *dualists*; that is, they think that the mind and the body are separate entities. Nietzsche is not a dualist, but a *monist*—which means that he thinks of the mind and the body as being the same thing.

Nietzsche and Atkins are in agreement: recall Atkins's remark that a fair percentage of alleged mental illness would vanish if only people would eat properly (p. 134).

Why is Nietzsche so concerned with the question of nutriment? Certainly a large part of his interest arises from his own poor health. However, it is precisely this poor health that he says drove him to reflect upon reason itself. Nietzsche as philosopher is chiefly concerned with the health of modern culture. His concern for the question of nutriment—which as I mentioned above is the question of how to how best to nourish oneself so as to attain a maximum of strength—is directed not only at physical vitality, but also at cultural vitality. By strength, Nietzsche means a particular kind of virtue, which he calls "moraline-free virtue" (*EH*, II, §1). This rather bizarre phrase, which sounds deeply paradoxical to a logical ear, actually starts to make quite a bit of sense if we think of Nietzsche as opposing a culture, and especially the values of a culture, that he thinks has grown weak, decadent, and unhealthy.

The Atkins Culture

Anyone who has ever tried, and failed, to lose weight is only too aware that certain alleged facts about nutrition just don't add up. "Eat more bread and pasta, because they fill you up" (they don't). "Losing weight is simply a matter of willpower" (if it were, we'd all be a size 6). "Low-fat foods taste just as good as the higher-fat version" (come on now, be serious!). It's not difficult to see how attractive an "alternative" diet such as Atkins can be, especially to those of us who love our food, and who have counted our low-fat calories with extraordinary patience, utter commitment, and—unfortunately—absolutely no success. Atkins claims to offer us an enjoyable, and a healthy, way of eating that will also enable us to lose weight and solve associated health problems. And thereby, Atkins offers us another chance to fit in—quite literally—with the expectations of contemporary culture, which of course include a slim and healthy appearance. Be honest, now: we have all heard of people who have lost out on jobs, promotions, relationships, family, self-respect—all things that are currently considered culturally important—because of excess weight. If we're really honest, we know that some of us are those people.

Atkins offers us an explanation for our weight problem coupled with a realistic potential solution to that problem. Serial dieters know that the most puzzling and frustrating thing for a dieter who fails to lose weight on a low-fat diet, assuming that one followed its rules diligently, is *why* one has failed. A common reaction is for the dieter, or the dieter's friends, family, and general practitioner, to blame the failure on a fault in willpower or dedication, even despite the dieter's awareness that the rules were followed correctly. According to Atkins, however, many of our weight-loss problems are metabolic and indeed cultural, rather than straightforwardly psychological. Atkins believes that our food culture has changed substantially following the introduction of aggressively mass-marketed foods that are heavily processed, and contain large quantities of refined sugar and preservative chemicals. These foods now dominate our culture in a way that was unimaginable only one hundred and fifty years ago. The way in which we think about our food, what we eat, and how we eat has changed dramatically in a comparatively short time; in many cases, Atkins claims, affecting our metabolic responses to carbohydrates (pp. 27, 44–46). Most of our food no longer has a high nutritional value; instead, we have replaced nutritious, natural foods such as fresh meat and vegetables with the nutritionally valueless, or empty, calories found in things like cakes and cookies (p. 28). We've come to believe that eating processed, mass-produced foods containing unnatural fats and chemicals is not only normal, but healthy. According to Atkins, this belief is making us sick.

There is a fascinating parallel to be drawn between Atkins's account of the degeneration of our food culture and Nietzsche's critique of modern culture. Nietzsche thinks that our culture has become nihilistic. Nihilism, put simply, is the philosophical view that there is there are no values, and that life is therefore worthless. Nietzsche thinks that our values have become meaningless, or devalued, over time. In the later nineteenth century, nihilistic attitudes were increasingly present within Western European culture, owing to the perceived decline of the dominant religion, Christianity.[5] Nietzsche's infamous announcement of the "death

[5] For more on the death of God and cultural therapy, see Robert Wicks, *Nietzsche* (Oxford: Oneworld, 2002).

of God," in *Thus Spoke Zarathustra* resulted from his conviction that a culture based on Christian values was sick—because the belief in God, he thought, was actually more detrimental to the health of culture than nonbelief.[6] Therefore, Nietzsche became convinced that modern culture requires therapy in order to regain its health. To put this more generally, Nietzsche thought that belief in God stands in direct opposition to a healthy life, and like a competent physician, his concern was to do something to protect and promote healthy life. Accepting the death of God is the first step in Nietzsche's therapeutic protocol.

Dr. Atkins's reason for setting out his diet is based on his reaction to what we might well call nutritional nihilism, and his solution requires that we change our whole way of thinking about what we eat. Nietzsche's critique of modern culture introduces us to the main aim of his wider philosophy: to restore modern culture to a state of health and vitality. Like Atkins's diet, Nietzsche's nutritional project of cultural revitalization requires that a number of our preconceptions about the world must be challenged.

Science and the Nietzsche Diet

Within the philosophy of science, methodology, which critically explores the methods by which science arrives at truths about the world, is most closely related to theories of knowledge and of truth.[7] In empirical science, natural phenomena are measured and described by observers who consciously set aside their individual beliefs, motives, and cultural backgrounds in order to produce properly objective empirical results and evaluations.[8] The defining strength of science is its value-freedom, which is derived from science's chief aim of an observer-independent account of the world that transcends human meaning, culture, and ideology. Though, of course, this is not to say that science

---

[6] Nietzsche, *Thus Spoke Zarathustra* (Harmondsworth: Penguin, 1969).

[7] See Lawrence Sklar, "Philosophy of Science," in Robert Audi, ed., *The Cambridge Dictionary of Philosophy* (Cambridge: Cambridge University Press, 1995), p. 611.

[8] Anthony O'Hear, "'Two Cultures' Revisited," *Verstehen and Humane Understanding: Royal Institute of Philosophy Supplement* 41 (Cambridge: Cambridge University Press, 1996), p. 4.

is oblivious to matters of human interest.[9] Through scientific method, the general claim is that we can come to know the way things really are in the world—in short, that science gives us truth. The view that empirical science gives us truths about the world seems uncontroversial to most people.

A responsible would-be Atkins dieter, wanting to make an informed decision as to whether or not to adopt the diet, might well look to modern science for proof of the diet's safety and efficacy for weight loss, and for evidence of its nutritional value. For Atkins, as we've seen, the main problem to overcome is that we don't really think about what we eat or how we eat it—and we certainly don't understand the enormous cultural shift that has taken place with respect to our attitudes towards our food. However, this can be as true of medical professionals, scientists, and dieticians as it is of ordinary folk. So asking a doctor or a nutritionist for advice on doing Atkins, or researching the topic for yourself, can produce a range of conflicting results, all of which seem to be backed up by scientific evidence. Atkins bemoans the type of "mega-orthodox" doctor who fails to appreciate the process of medicine but instead simply worships the conclusions of medical consensus with "religious fervor" (p. 144). Atkins's problem with medical consensus is that, unlike him, it ignores empirical evidence in favor of prevailing opinion (p. 73).

Atkins's concern about medical consensus echoes some of Nietzsche's views on science. In *Twilight of the Idols*, which narrowly precedes *Ecce Homo*, Nietzsche claims that nihilism is a direct product of degeneration of the mind in its relation to culture over time (*TI* 8, §§ 2, 3).[10] As evidence of this, Nietzsche points out that "*passion* in intellectual matters is going more and more downhill" (*TI* 8, §3), and he laments that the sciences have been de-intellectualized. The previously healthy state of the life of the mind has been made sick by, and through, nihilistic culture. But here we come to more of a distinction between Nietzsche and Atkins on the subject of science. Atkins claims that while empirical science is objec-

---

[9] *Ibid.*, pp. 3–5.

[10] Throughout, I use the standard abbreviation *TI* for Nietzsche's *Twilight of the Idols*. I have used the translation by Duncan Large (Oxford: Oxford University Press, 1998).

tive and value-free, some professionals give more credence to consensus than to plain scientific facts. Atkins therefore keeps to the scientific faith. Nietzsche, however, is less convinced of the overweening value of science. In his first published book, *The Birth of Tragedy*, he became the first philosopher to raise what he calls the problem of science—specifically, to consider the notion of science itself as problematic and questionable.[11]

For Nietzsche, a therapeutic responsibility to question science exists precisely because science dominates our thinking in modern culture. Put simply, Nietzsche thinks that our modern tendency to resort to science in all matters creates an imbalance in modern culture, and thereby contributes to its unhealthy state. In a sense, scientific truths act as a replacement for divine truth in the wake of God's death. As such, when understood as a cultural value, science simply stands in for religious value—and hence science itself becomes an expression of cultural nihilism. But this attitude towards science doesn't mean that Nietzsche is antiscience *per se*—and indeed, Nietzsche became increasingly interested in science during his life.[12] The point is that it's our way of thinking—and specifically, our lack of thinking—that causes the problem.

The "Truth" of the Atkins Matter

As we've seen, developed-world culture relies heavily upon modern science to provide solutions to all of its problems—or at least to provide explanations as to why these problems exist. Contemporary nutritional advice is based on scientific evidence. For example, in order to defend and justify the diet's nutritional recommendations, the Atkins Foundation funds scientific studies into the long-term effects of low-carbohydrate eating and any demonstrable associated health benefits, and even makes some of these directly available to dieters through publications and through the Atkins Center website. Not to be left out, critics of Atkins, especially those who are medical-nutrition professionals,

---

[11] Nietzsche, *The Birth of Tragedy* (1872) (Harmondsworth: Penguin, 1993).

[12] See Babette E. Babich, *Nietzsche's Philosophy of Science: Reflecting Science on the Ground of Art and Life* (Albany: State University of New York Press, 1994).

refer to a range of scientific evidence in order to drive their point home: support for Atkins depends on poor, or scanty, science. However, reliance upon science can also cause problems. As we've seen, Nietzsche thinks that science itself can be an expression of nihilism, when it's taken as a cultural value. Instead of a set of values that grounds a culture and defines what is true and what is permitted, nihilism, as construed by a culture in nihilistic crisis, is the notion that nothing is true and that everything is permitted.[13]

Let's get down to the big question: to do Atkins, or not to do Atkins? Answering this question isn't as easy as we might think. First of all, how are we supposed to know exactly how Atkins works, whether or not Atkins works, and whether or not Atkins is really any good for us? On which, or whose, criteria are we supposed to base the decisions about which nutritional advice to follow that our culture increasingly forces us to make? If a potential dieter is to get to the truth of the Atkins matter, in order to make an informed decision, then turning to science alone isn't going to help them. As Atkins points out, epidemiological studies can cast significant doubt upon, say, the hypothesis that high-fat diets cause heart disease—but these studies don't actually prove anything (p. 197). Between the publications of his *Diet Revolution* and *New Diet Revolution*, Atkins claims that a number of studies supporting the insights of low-carbohydrate diets have emerged (p. 9). However, none of these actually tell us, once and for all, what the truth of the matter is. None of them are able to do so, for the following reason: scientific experimentation cannot escape its inductive nature. Especially where human nutrition is concerned, empirical evidence simply isn't capable of adding up to much—there are so many variables at work that the inductive inference upon which any empirical claim is dependent remains essentially weak. Put simply, it's phenomenally difficult to make any general, empirical claims about the nutritional needs of human beings. This is why Atkins must ask us to think about our food culture for ourselves, and to make our own decision about whether or not to choose a low-carbohydrate lifestyle. Although he believes that low-carbohydrate eating is the natural human diet, he allows for human

---

[13] See Ofelia Schutte, *Beyond Nihilism: Nietzsche without Masks* (Chicago: University of Chicago Press, 1984).

biological individuality, freely acknowledging that the diet is not for everyone (p. 28).

The same individualism is present in Nietzsche's critique of truth. Traditional theories of truth work on a correspondence model, in which, for example, the proposition that snow is white is true by virtue of its correspondence to a feature of the external world, namely the whiteness of snow.[14] Unlike Atkins, however, Nietzsche does not have much faith in objective truth; instead, he offers us a critique of truth that challenges our belief in the existence of facts, and a new theory of truth, perspectivism, based on interpretation. In allowing that there are no uninterpreted facts or truths, Nietzsche is not simply claiming that all facts are really interpretations, but is arguing in a deeper sense that only the interpretation is "real."[15] In *Human, All Too Human*, Nietzsche argues that "we behold all things through the human head and cannot cut off this head" (§27).[16] He defines the human perspective in terms of the link between interpretation and the organic. The implication of this assessment is that we cannot divorce evaluative judgments from our various physiological perspectives. The designation of something as a fact integrally involves the imposition of value. The idea is that we cannot separate that which is construed as "fact" from interpretation—we cannot subtract the human element from the determination of the fact.

Nietzsche thinks that our belief in truth acts in the same way as our belief in science and our belief in God. Unreflective faith in truth, science, and religion all contribute to the nihilistic crisis in modern culture. Hence he emphasizes the importance of interpretation in order to counterbalance the cultural effect of our belief in truth. From a Nietzschean perspective, thinking about "the truth" of the Atkins matter makes no sense because there is no real, objective truth to be had. There are only interpretations, and we are all accountable for these. So responsible would-be dieters must, on a Nietzschean account, take on the full burden

[14] Paul Horwich, "Theories of Truth," in Jaegwon Kim and Ernest Sosa, eds., *A Companion to Metaphysics* (Oxford: Blackwell, 1995), p. 492.

[15] Alan D. Schrift, *Nietzsche and the Question of Interpretation: Between Hermeneutics and Deconstruction,* (New York: Routledge, 1990), p. 151.

[16] Nietzsche, *Human, All Too Human* (Harmondsworth: Penguin, 1994).

of responsibility for their own nutrition. The truth of the Atkins matter, from a Nietzschean perspective, is generated through interpretation from the individual's physiological perspective.

Lifetime Maintenance: Nietzsche's Healthy Culture

Nietzsche's critiques of science and truth, which some consider unbalanced, aim towards achieving a balanced result. Nietzsche does not, as is sometimes thought, devalue science and truth entirely. Instead, he places them into an appropriate cultural context. If we are to return to, and sustain, a healthy culture, Nietzsche thinks we must ensure that interpretation and value creation take center stage in our lives. Adopting a Nietzschean approach can help us to realize the cultural importance of making our own interpretations of small (or occasionally rather large) matters, such as nutritional advice. As we have seen, Dr. Atkins's dietary approach has a good deal in common with Nietzsche. Atkins's greatest asset lies in acceptance of human biological individuality. It is on this basis that Atkins encourages us to experiment with the diet and to interpret our results for ourselves, while also acknowledging that the diet may not be right for everyone. He thereby encourages us to take an individualistic approach to the broader question of human nutrition. Dr. Atkins prescribes an unbalanced corrective diet for an unbalanced modern metabolism. The result, he hopes, is a balanced one—or at least one which is in proportion with its height and build!

Still, Atkins and Nietzsche differ on the issue of science. Where Nietzsche feels it necessary to question the overweening value of science as a part of his project of cultural therapy, Atkins remains convinced that science can offer a definitive answer to the question of nutrition. Could the Atkins recipe for a healthy food culture perhaps benefit from a dash more Nietzsche? Atkins Nutritionals' ongoing mass-marketing of processed, low-carbohydrate foods, and the paeans recently offered to the low-fat/health consensus by the Atkins Foundation, seem to cut against the grain of Dr. Atkins's original thinking. As we saw, Atkins's books emphasized the need for a change in our food culture in the form of a rejection of nutritional nihilism through the reclamation of a natural approach to nutrition, based on scientific evidence supporting these views. But regardless of its implementation by Dr. Atkins or by the corporate, charitable, and research institutions arising from his work, the Atkins difference remains vulnerable to the belief that there is a definitive answer to a general question of optimal human nutrition, and that this answer is generated, and can be verified, empirically. Following Nietzsche, authentic cultural therapy aimed at overcoming nihilism demands that we question all of our presuppositions and values—including those that concern modern science. If Dr. Atkins had taken a properly Nietzschean route, he would have been required to give up his absolute faith in empirical science in order to lend sufficient weight to his claims concerning the role of individual interpretation in human nutrition. This faith was not something that he could afford to give up. Can any of us do any better? On this point and on many others, much as both Nietzsche and Dr. Atkins advise, doing better is making our own decisions (p. 205).

9

The Structure of Atkins's New Diet Revolution: Proposing a Paradigm Shift in Fighting Obesity

CATHERINE A. WOMACK

The Weighty Problem of Obesity in America

The Atkins Diet offers a lifeline for an America sinking under its own weight. We all know the bad news. The National Institute of Diabetes and Digestive and Kidney Diseases[1] provides us with the following sobering statistics: 64 percent of Americans are overweight. More than 30 percent of Americans are also obese. Obesity is responsible for more than 300,000 preventable deaths each year in the United States, second only to smoking. The epidemic has affected children as well; 15 percent of children under eighteen are obese, and another 15 percent are overweight. Why is this happening?[2] Most health experts point to sedentary lifestyles and diets that include mostly energy-dense (high-fat, high-sugar, high-calorie) food. In short, we consume too much and exercise too little.

---

[1] Weight Control Information Network: An Information Service of the National Institutes of Diabetes and Digestive and Kidney Diseases (NIDDK); Statistics Related to Overweight and Obesity: http://win.niddk.nih.gov/statistics/index .htm. Hereafter cited as NIDDK, 2004.

[2] These sources are helpful on this subject: Adam Benforado, Jon Hanson, and David Yosifon, "Broken Scales: Obesity and Justice in America," *Emory Law Journal* 53 (2004), p. 1645; Kelly D. Brownell and Katherine Battle Horgen, *Food Fight: The Inside Story of the Food Industry, America's Obesity Crisis, and What We Can Do About It* (New York: McGraw-Hill, 2003); Ellen Ruppel Shell, *The Hungry Gene: The Science of Fat and the Future of Thin* (New York: Atlantic Monthly Press, 2002); Mimi Spencer, "Let Them Eat Cake," *The*

And there's more bad news. Try as we might and spend as we do on weight loss programs and products—$33 billion a year—almost all Americans who diet fail to keep the weight off (NIDDK, 2004). Many, if not most, dieters regain all they had lost and then some, so that the result of their dieting efforts is that they are fatter than when they started.

This seems like a simple problem with a simple solution. If excess calorie intake is the problem, then we should simply reduce the number of calories we consume and work to burn more of them. In short, we should eat less and exercise more. But as we know, diets are very hard to follow, and big lifestyle changes are even harder to maintain over the long term.

The Atkins Diet offers us something that we thought impossible: a way to lose weight and not feel deprived and starved while losing. Atkins (and its kinder, gentler cousin, the South Beach diet) offer a shift in our old dieting paradigm—a new way of thinking about eating and weight loss. The advice turns conventional dieting wisdom upside down. It's not calories but carbohydrates that are responsible for obesity, says Atkins: By restricting carbohydrates, the body, through a process called ketosis, allegedly burns more fat. Also, the restriction of carbs reduces food cravings so dieters will eat less. Consuming more fat and protein leaves dieters feeling more satisfied, so they will be able to stay on the diet for the longer term.

The Atkins Diet represents a potential shift in the accepted scientific view about weight loss. In all areas of science, shifts do sometimes occur as researchers make significant new discoveries. Before the seventeenth century, much of the scientific community practiced astronomy that relied on the idea of an earth-centered solar system. Ptolemaic astronomy—named after Greek astronomer Ptolemy (who lived from approxiamately A.D. 85 to approxiamately A.D. 165), who developed the theory—the prevailing science of the heavens, placed the Earth as the center of the cosmos. However, there were many problems with this view, including the fact that much of the data collected by scientists seemed to contradict the theory. Ptolemaic geocentric (earth-centered) theory was replaced by a heliocentric (sun-centered) theory put forth by the Polish astronomer Nicholas

---

Observer (7th November, 2004), http://observer.guardian.co.uk/foodmonthly/story/0,9950,1342296,00.html.

Copernicus (1473–1543). According to Copernican theory, the sun is at the center of the solar system, with the planets (including the Earth) rotating around it in elliptical orbits. The seventeenth-century astronomer Galileo was instrumental in bringing about the shift to the Copernican theory; his work combined theory and observation, and he developed early telescopes to make more detailed observations possible. Adoption of the Copernican theory was a major shift in scientists' view of the universe.

Philosopher Thomas Kuhn described such drastic shifts in our scientific world views as "paradigm shifts." In his influential 1962 book *The Structure of Scientific Revolutions*, Kuhn set out to explain how science changes and progresses. He argued that, instead of progressing cumulatively, adding to our stockpile of knowledge, science progresses through the development and overthrow of paradigms. We can think of a paradigm as a set of scientific practices (including development of laws, applications, instruments, and so on) that "provide models from which spring particular coherent traditions of scientific research."[3] When a scientist achieves success in solving a fundamental problem, attracts other scientists to her research program, and sets the stage for further expansion of research in her field, she has established a paradigm. Copernicus, Newton, and Lavoisier are a few of the scientists whose achievements served to define the problems and methods of a research field for many generations (Kuhn, p. 10). Paradigms bring together scientists with shared assumptions about the relevant phenomena to be explored, the most interesting problems to tackle, and the best methods to use.

In astronomy, the paradigm shift from Ptolemaic to Copernican theory was gradual; the idea that the earth was moving through space seemed false given our experience of a stable planet. But over time, evidence began to mount: about a century after Copernicus proposed the theory, the telescope came into use, allowing for more extensive and accurate data collection on planetary and star movement. Even later, new mathematics was developed that both made the theory clearer and resulted in solutions to problems previously considered too

[3] Thomas Kuhn, *The Structure of Scientific Revolutions* (Chicago: University of Chicago Press, 1962), p. 10.

difficult. A paradigm requires time and a variety of sources of confirmation to get a foothold; once there is a record of successful research based on it, it becomes more fully established.

The focus on individual diets as the best approach to long-term weight loss can be seen as an example of a paradigm. One of the marks of a paradigm is that it identifies certain features of a phenomenon as the crucial ones to explore, and ignores other features as unimportant. Even though there are many disparate causes of obesity, medical science has settled on individual behaviors as the most important causes (ignoring, for the most part, environmental or socioeconomic factors). That's why doctors and nutritionists focus on diets as the way to address obesity. The main research program of the diet paradigm is to find the right combination of types and amounts of foods that individuals can eat so that they will lose weight and maintain weight loss. Virtually all programs also add in regular physical activity—another individual behavior.

Although obesity-reduction programs all focus on dieting as the best way to achieve long-term weight loss, there is no consensus on which particular diet is most effective. Experts have shifted their support from low-fat to high-protein to restricted-calorie to low-carb and back again. The Atkins Diet has enjoyed a recent surge of popularity even among many experts, spawning research into the relationship between carbohydrates, fats, protein, calories, and body weight. However, in order for Atkins to take the lead as the primary program providing support for the dieting paradigm, it needs both to attract researchers to its program and to demonstrate major progress in bringing about successful weight loss. Has Atkins got what it takes to provide crucial support for the dieting paradigm? I don't think so. I think the dieting paradigm itself is flawed and should be replaced with a new paradigm that proposes to address problems of obesity by focusing on the community, not the individual. More on this later, but first, let's see what Kuhn has to say about how paradigms work.

Paradigms for Heavenly and Earthly Bodies

Kuhn's work aims at understanding how big research programs in the sciences develop and gain strength over time, and what causes the downfall and replacement of those programs.

Understanding the general process can help us see how it applies to the science of dieting.

Kuhn argues that science progresses through a number of phases. As people start to investigate nature, they start identifying particular phenomena as the crucial ones for understanding how the world works. At some point in the past, astronomers noticed that the night sky changed in appearance over the course of days, weeks, and months. This suggested that the heavenly bodies (whatever they were) moved across the sky. As people shared their work based on a sun-centered solar system, some of them made real achievements not possible from within the Ptolemaic system—they were able to predict the motions of the bodies, they developed theories to explain their motions—resulting in a clearer, more consistent view of what the universe was like. In this way, the Copernican astronomical paradigm became established. Paradigms, says Kuhn, "gain their status because they are more successful than their competitors in solving a few problems that the group of practitioners has come to recognize as acute" (Kuhn, p. 23). Using the Copernican paradigm, Galileo was able to put together better solutions to problems, extend the theory, and develop new instruments (like the telescope) to better understand the motions of the stars and planets.

Kuhn says that paradigms provide ways to select research problems from all the possibilities—to focus on certain features of a phenomenon as important and to ignore other features as less important. Even though there are many causes of obesity, current approaches center on ways to regulate the food intake of individuals through specifying the appropriate combinations and amounts. Work within the dieting paradigm revealed links between fat intake and heart disease, for instance. Low-carb diets helped spur research on connections between carbohydrate intake and insulin resistance, a condition considered by many as a precursor to Type-II diabetes.

Kuhn uses the term "normal science" to refer to mainstream scientific research within a paradigm. This type of research was based on scientific achievements considered foundational by the scientific community. Kuhn says that research based on a common paradigm involves a commitment to the same rules and standards for scientific practice (Kuhn, p. 11). Unfortunately, the science of dieting is less advanced than astronomy; we know more about the behavior of the stars than about human metabolism. As a result, researchers have not been very successful in solving their main problem: how to control obesity.

However, there are some shared assumptions among food scientists. They have included classifying the four basic food groups, which were replaced by the familiar food pyramid. Some basic assumptions that guide dieting practices are that we should eat a variety of foods, and that carbohydrates should constitute a large percentage of our food intake. Fats should constitute a small percentage of our diet because they have been linked to heart disease and other serious health problems.

Atkins challenges these assumptions, and turns the food pyramid (almost) upside down. Does it represent an important shift within the dieting paradigm for understanding how we should eat in order to be healthy? In order to do so it must have a record of success in solving the paradigm's main problem, namely bringing about long-term weight loss. Let's see what the research says.

Rating the Effectiveness of the Low-Carb Paradigm: A Scientific Report Card

Within a paradigm, researchers agree on some standard problems to solve. Any dieting paradigm will have as one of its main problems the design of a diet that (1) results in weight loss; (2) helps people keep weight off over time; (3) is reasonably practical to follow for most people; and (4) has no significant negative effects on overall health.

As we know, diet researchers have made little progress on any of these fronts. Kuhn explained that the recognition of failures within normal science is very important for scientific progress. He used the term "anomaly" to refer to phenomena that show our research goals are not being met; somehow, nature is thwarting the expectations that have been set up within the paradigm. Anomalies help trigger changes in assumptions and pave the way for shifts and eventual overthrow of paradigms. The apparent effectiveness, at least in the short term, of low-carb diets seems to present an anomaly for the standard diet paradigm, as it violates shared assumptions about restrictions on calorie and fat intake. But is Atkins really effective? Does it present a genuine anomaly for the standard diet paradigm?

Let's start with (1) and (2): short- and long-term weight loss. Many studies show Atkins dieters losing more weight in the first three to six months than their low-fat dieting counterparts do. In one survey of medical studies comparing moderately obese low-carb dieters to low-fat dieters, researchers found that at six months the low-carb group lost on average eight to twelve pounds more than the low-fat group. However, at the twelve-month mark the weight losses for the groups were about the same: less than a five-pound difference between groups.[4] In a recent study comparing one-year weight losses for Atkins with the Ornish, Zone, and Weight Watchers diets, researchers found no significant differences between the groups, and only modest (five to eight pounds) average weight losses after one year.[5] More studies need to be done, but so far it does not look as if Atkins delivers either the drastic short-term or the enduring long-term weight loss it promises. Of course, neither do the other diets. We see two sorts of data here: (1) Atkins seems to produce short-term weight loss and some improvement in risk factors for heart disease and diabetes, suggesting that the shift is warranted; (2) unfortunately, when we look at long-term weight loss, no diets (including Atkins) are effective.

Measuring the practicality of a diet is not easy. One way scientists do this is to count how many people in a medical study drop out and how many who stay in actually stick to the diet. What they find is both a high dropout rate—anywhere from 30 to 50 percent in a survey of ten recent studies on low-carb diets, and low adherence rates—fewer than 60 percent stick to the diet prescribed (Obesity Online, 2004). Even though anecdotes from successful Atkins dieters are common, the overall statistics are not good; many if not most people either give up dieting altogether or cheat their way back to weight gain.

What about the effects of low-carb dieting on health? Atkins and the South Beach diets promise lowered cholesterol and blood-glucose levels, which suggests that they help people

---

[4] Obesity Online. 2004. Slide on weight loss at six months of low-fat vs. low-carb diets. http://www.obesityonline.org/slides/slide01.cfm?q=and+hdl-cholesterol&dpg=2.

[5] Michael L. Dansinger, M.D., *et al.* "Comparison of the Atkins, Ornish, Weight Watchers, and Zone Diets for Weight Loss and Heart Disease Risk Reduction: A Randomized Trial." *Journal of the American Medical Association* 293, no. 1 (2005), pp. 43–53.

decrease their risks both for cardiovascular disease and Type-II diabetes. In several medical studies this seems to be confirmed: in comparison with other diets, Atkins either matches or beats them in lowered cholesterol, blood glucose, and blood pressure levels. However, many researchers believe that the patterns of high-fat intake will increase risks for heart disease. Also, there are worries about possible correlations between high protein intake and compromised kidney functioning. Everyone agrees that long-term studies are needed to measure the health effects over time of low-carb diets.

So, it looks as if Atkins does not present a significant anomaly for the standard dieting paradigm; it seems to be no more successful than other diets at long-term weight loss, and it's unclear whether the associated health risks and benefits make it a safer alternative to standard low-fat or low-calorie diets.

Dieting in Crisis: What to Do When Paradigms Fail

We've so far seen research that suggests that the Atkins Diet is no more successful than any other diet. Even worse, no diet has been shown successful in helping achieve long-term weight loss; few dieters maintain any weight loss at all after five years. Kuhn would describe this situation as a crisis for the dieting paradigm. There are anomalies everywhere in the form of studies that show no appreciable weight loss over time, no matter what sort of diet is pursued. What this means is that the basic research programs have been a dismal failure; even shifts within the paradigm to alternatives like low-carb, low-fat, and very low-calorie have yielded no discernible long-term results.

With respect to the diet as weight-loss tool, we're in a state of crisis. Kuhn described crisis in this way: even though we are still committed to the paradigm, no one agrees either exactly what it is or whether it is solving any of the problems we think are important. We are all still searching for a solution to the obesity problem by focusing on what individuals put on their plates. But, there is no general agreement on what combination of foods is the right one for weight loss. How do we resolve this crisis? Again, Kuhn has some advice, describing three ways scientific crises can come to a close.

First, normal science may prove able to handle the crisis-provoking problem, thus saving the paradigm. Maybe someone will discover the perfect combination of foods that will produce weight loss and be satisfying and manageable. However, no candidates are on the horizon. Gastric bypass surgery is gaining in popularity as a solution for the increasing ranks of those desperate for weight control; they turn to surgery despite our ignorance of its long-term success rate and its effects on health.

Second, maybe the crisis-producing problem will resist even radical new approaches, so we conclude that no solution is forthcoming; we then set the problem aside to await the tools of future generations. This does not seem like an option, especially given the epidemic of obesity-related illnesses among adults and children. Waiting around for new technology or different approaches is a luxury we cannot afford.

So, we arrive at the third option: the crisis may end with the emergence of a new paradigm, with a fundamentally different world view and new problem-solving methods.

Replacing the Dieting Paradigm: A Radical Shift from the Plate to the Environment

If diets don't work—not even Atkins—then what options do we have in our fight against obesity? Everyone knows we should eat fewer brownies and more celery. But, it's just too hard for us to make the celery-over-brownies choice once they are on the plate. What should we do instead? I think we should look outward to see what environmental factors make it harder for us to pick celery over brownies. In this way we shift away from causes of obesity at the level of the individual and towards external causes in our communities. What we need here is a new paradigm to replace the failed diet one.

Some experts are looking in unusual places for these external factors—France, for example. There have been many articles in recent years about the so-called French Paradox—the French eat very rich, fat-laden foods and do not exercise a lot, yet they have the lowest obesity rates (less than 10 percent) in Europe. What are they doing right?[6]

[6] One book that discusses the French paradox is Mireille Guiliano, *French Women Don't Get Fat: The Secret of Eating for Pleasure* (New York: Knopf, 2004).

Here's a possible answer: the French live in a culture in which people do not eat processed or fast food. They take time to eat their meals, and they enjoy their food. French people are more active in their daily lives and less car-dependent than Americans.

We Americans, however, eat fast food and processed food in large quantities. The food we eat is loaded with fat and sugar. Most of us live in communities where we have to drive to mail a letter, buy groceries, or get a cup of coffee. When we do get in our cars, we run the gauntlet of fast-food joints, all beckoning us with low-priced, instantly available high-calorie foods that we have become used to eating regularly.

Public health experts are writing about our "toxic food environment" and what to do about it. Many argue that obesity is a public health problem, not an individual medical one. What they are advocating is overthrowing the diet paradigm and replacing it with a community-based paradigm as a way to address the problem of obesity. By shifting the focus away from diets and towards the community in which the individual lives, it may be possible to create an environment in which healthy eating and lifestyle habits are easier to establish and maintain over time.

For instance, everyone knows that regular physical activity is key to maintaining a healthy weight. If I live in a neighborhood with no sidewalks and lots of busy streets with no pedestrian crosswalks, it will be much harder for me to take that daily walk in the morning or after dinner. Seeing the problem from a community viewpoint can reveal new solutions—citizens' groups can organize and lobby for bike paths or zoning laws to encourage more mixed-use areas where people can live and shop in the same place. This new paradigm works on a larger scale as well: for instance, if states with interstate highway rest stops replaced fast food vendors with healthier food outlets, it would be easier for travelers to maintain healthy eating habits on the road.

These new problems are very difficult and complex ones. According to Kuhn, in order for the new paradigm to become entrenched, we will have to develop new tools for problem-solving and use them successfully over time. I think that community organizing and lobbying for government regulation are promising methods. This works at many levels, from starting a neighborhood dog-walking group to lobbying Congress to regulate food advertising targeted at children.

Obesity is an epidemic that we must address; the economic and human costs are enormous. By shifting the focus to the external and environmental causes of obesity, we open up many new avenues of research, advocacy, and control. There are many ways for us to take control of our health, fitness, and sense of self worth. Diets promise us the world and produce feelings of failure and hopelessness. If we accept that the failure is in them and not us, then we can move on to find new ways of shaping our communities, and through them, our own lives.

Part 4

Vitamins and Minerals

(Socio-political and Ethical Considerations)

10
Commodious Diets, or Could a Marxist Do Atkins?

BAT-AMI BAR ON

Laying the Groundwork for a Lifetime of Health

I like food. Because I grew up in Israel, my tastes are rather Mediterranean. When I first heard about the Atkins Diet, as well as other relatively low-carb diets such as the South Beach diet, I felt an immediate sense of deprivation since a low-carb diet rules out the breads and pasta that are the staples of my diet, the hummus and many other bean dishes I savor, let alone the desserts and chocolates that I like to eat quite often. So at face value, to me, low-carb diets should seem quite unappealing. But, I also, at various times, try to lose a bit of weight. Tastes aside, I am vain enough and prefer to look trimmer and more fit, so diets that offer that possibility, especially when they also promise quick results, are liable to intrigue me. Therefore, I recently checked the Atkins Diet website and also the Atkins's competitor, the South Beach diet website.[1]

The Atkins website is the more interesting of the two, though both sites advertise a low-carb diet. One of the things that makes the Atkins Diet website more interesting is that it presents the same thing—the Atkins Diet—in several packages, each designed for a specific target audience. The last time I checked, the website identified one target audience as consisting of four

---

[1] I was reading these pages (http://Atkins.com and http://www.southbeachdiet.com/public/default.asp) in December 2004.

mainly English speaking countries—the United States (the diet's home country), Australia, Canada, and the United Kingdom. Another target audience was Latin American, addressed as one Spanish-speaking audience, despite the many cultural variations one can find in Latin America. The target audience in Brazil was addressed separately in Portuguese. The website addresses additional target audiences in the Netherlands, Norway, and Sweden in the most common of the local languages.

As I examined the first pages for these varied target audiences and noticed the care with which the Atkins Diet is packaged, I began to wonder about the kind of commodity that this diet is. Diets do not seem like commodities and it might be the case that not all diets are commodities. But, the Atkins Diet is a commodity.

A *commodity* is a product that is sold in some market to buyers with specific preferences. However, this definition-like statement regarding the nature of commodities simplifies too much. This will become clear later especially after I turn to Marx. When I reflect upon commodities, I like to turn to Marx for help since he was among the first systematic critical analysts of commodities, and thus among the first to expose the complexity of commodities.

Karl Marx (1818–1883) did not invent the term "commodity." According to the *Oxford English Dictionary*, the English word "commodity" is related etymologically to the French word "commodité," which was used in the fifteenth century and means fitness, convenience, or complaisance, and refers to the quality or condition of things in relation to human desire or need. Commodities accommodate us, or more precisely, we perceive them to do so. The difference between actually accommodating and being perceived as accommodating is very important.

Being accommodating is a possible feature or attribute of something just like being blue or being salty are. Since perception is not necessarily veridical or accurate and can be erroneous and misleading, when something is perceived as possessing some characteristic, such as being accommodating, it is sensible to ask whether the characteristic is real. Does the thing in question actually have the characteristic that it is perceived to have, namely, is it actually accommodating? In the case of a diet, any diet, as one ponders the possible gap between what is real and what merely appears to be real, one may want to find out *how* and *what* it accommodates. What are the needs that it is supposed to fulfill? Why are there such needs? Does it promise better health? Does it promise a look? Does it work, for what exactly does it work, and does it work long-term as a food regimen?

These questions are important since diets appeal to people for many reasons and they tend to fail unless they are already the diet one follows, that is, one's usual food regimen or pattern, rather than the diet one is "on." Some diets are culturally patterned, though globalization is changing this rapidly by making many culture-specific foods available everywhere. Some diets are healthier than others. Various experts are now touting the so-called "Mediterranean diet."[2] While a misnomer because there are many Mediterranean diets rather than a single one, the "Mediterranean diet" is, nonetheless a culture-based diet that has developed over hundreds and even thousands of years. It is the food regimen of many people who grow up with it and not a diet to be "on," though it is beginning to be advertised and sold as a diet that one should be "on." Most diets that are advertised as diets one should be "on" are quite different from culturally-based food regimens with which people are raised no matter how good or bad they might be for one's health or looks.

The U.S. Department of Agriculture (USDA), which is responsible for the development and publications of guidelines for healthy eating for residents of the United States, revised its old guidelines in 2004.[3] It now recommends a diet that includes a variety of foods (to maximize nutritional intake), is calorically balanced (so that caloric intake is offset by caloric expenditure), is low in fats of all kinds, and exhibits moderation in the consumption of sugars, salts, and alcohol. The USDA-recommended diet recognizes that eating is pleasurable but insists that eating ought to be healthy and that there is no contradiction between the two. This is, of course, not obvious, especially given people's dietary habits. As William Grimes notes in "Eating My Spinach: Four Days on Uncle Sam's Diet," having decided to try to eat along the lines that the USDA recommends because he

---

[2] See http://www.trincoll.edu/~jvillani/Mediterranean.htm, or http://www.eufic.org/gb/food/pag/food43/food434.html (accessed December 2004).

[3] http://www.nal.usda.gov/fnic/dga/dguide95.html (accessed December 2004).

believed that would be easy for him, he began breaking the rules by the second day and found it impossible to stay on the USDA-recommended diet no matter how hard he tried. He did not think that he would fail so badly, since he thought at first that he had little in common with the people who really have to watch what they eat.[4]

Grimes suggests that his failure, which was a function of misjudgment, has a lot to do with American food culture. Thus, Grimes notes, given his own experience, that the USDA is recommending a cultural revolution, a radical change of eating patterns for the whole population.

Grimes's example with the USDA guidelines illustrates the difference between a diet one has and a diet to be "on," a difference that can go so far as to stand in extreme tension with one's ordinary way of life. As a result of this difference, a diet that one is to go "on" must have a certain appearance so as to be attractive to people who would not, due to their customs and routine practices, usually gravitate to it. It has to attract them despite themselves, despite their sense of who they are, and to do so it has to appear to them in a certain light. In the United States, the allure of diets is presumed to be connected to health or looks or both, especially if they seem to be related in such a way as to promise youthfulness too. Since most diets to be "on" are sold like all other commodities, the promise of better health and better looks (and youthfulness) is their hook. "Diets come and go, but what people hope to get from them remains fairly constant," declares the Atkins Diet web page. It goes on to claim: "With Atkins, you'll get the results you've dreamed of, without the agony of deprivation." And what you get is the rebalancing of "your nutrition so that you improve your energy level and your appearance and gain a sense of well-being. Following this approach lays the groundwork for a lifetime of better health."[5] This is the Atkins promise of how it will accommodate its possible consumers.

---

[4] William Grimes, "Eating My Spinach: Four Days on Uncle Sam's Diet," Week in Review, *New York Times* (23rd January, 2005). Also at http://www.nytimes.com/2005/01/23/weekinreview/23grim.html (accessed January 2005).

[5] http://atkins.com/Archive/2001/11/29-367514.html (accessed January 2005).

Need It, Want It, Got to Have It

The Atkins Diet is actually not exactly one commodity but several, a set of co-ordinated products manufactured and sold by a privately-owned commercial company called Atkins Nutritionals. According to *Hoover's*, the company began under a slightly different name in 1989 and now sells 250 "food products" such as power bars, nearly 100 nutritional supplements (such as essential oils) and "information products" such as books. These products are available at more than 30,000 stores,[6] and are also sold on the web. At present, the future of Atkins Nutiritionals is uncertain. On 5th December, 2004, the *New York Times* had a lengthy article about the slowing down of the low-carb business. The article pointed out that Atkins Nutritionals is feeling this slowdown—its revenues declined from $87 million in January of 2004 to $29 million in August—leading to speculations about the possibility that the company may have to default on debts, a fate which it had been trying to avoid by laying off 40 percent of its workforce.[7]

The decline in the sales of Atkins products points to customers' disenchantment. There are fewer people entering the market with an interest in acquiring this specific commodity. This may be because, like all fabricated diets, the Atkins Diet fails unless people actually change their lifestyles, and people have begun to realize this. Alternatively the decline is a function of critics having convinced people that the diet cannot deliver on its promises long term and may actually be unhealthy.[8] These explanations suggest that consumers, while having the same needs (for food and drink) and desires (for health, looks, and youthfulness), are not finding in the Atkins Diet the value they thought it might have. They do not perceive it as accommodating them, so it does not have the same value, utility, or "use-value" for them.

---

6 http://www.hoovers.com/atkins-nutritionals,-inc./—ID__115940—/free-co-factsheet.xhtml (accessed February 2005).

7 Melanie Warner, "Is the Low-Carb Boom Over: As Sales Slows, Atkins and Others Suffer," *The New York Times*, Section 3 (Business) (5th December, 2004), pp. 1, 9.

8 For an example of critical appraisals of the Atkins Diet see *Good Medicine* at http://www.pcrm.org/magazine/gm04SpringSummer/gm04SpringSummer01.html (accessed February 2005).

Commodities are assumed to have a "use-value." This is what perceiving them as able to respond to some need or desire means. So, when a commodity accommodates it has a "use-value." It not only has a "use-value," in Marx's terminology it *is* a "use-value," since a commodity accommodates because of its qualities (for example, a healthy diet has items that are indeed healthy to eat, like olive oil). A commodity's failure to accommodate means that it is lacking in "use-value" qualities, the qualities that make it useful. But then, something paradoxical happens since the item in question is not a commodity any more: it no longer meets the criteria for being a commodity. It does not accommodate. It is merely a product manufactured for a market with the hope that it can be sold and thus become a commodity. Or so it should be.

There are several reasons why the unsold product may still be, or at least may still appear to be, a commodity. For Marx this is the case because of a chain that begins with the familiar, namely the fact that "[a] commodity is, in the first place, an object outside us, a thing that by its properties satisfies human wants."[9] "The utility of a thing makes it a use-value" and in capitalist society use-values are "the material depositories of exchange-value."[10] It is due to its use-value that something can be put on a market to be sold to a buyer. The selling and buying are an exchange in which some commodity changes owners in exchange for money. Unlike use-values, which inhere in the commodity or are intrinsic to it and express a relation between a product and people's desires, exchange-values, belonging to commodities insofar as they are placed in a capitalist market, express a relation between commodities.

Money is perhaps the most exemplary of capitalist commodities. It has only exchange-value and its kind of exchange-value smoothes out whatever qualitative differences there may be among commodities when considered from the perspective of use-values, hence their unique qualities and their relations to people's desires. A book, a food product, a nutritional supplement—the basic elements of the marketed Atkins Diet—all have a price articulated in some monetary denomination that has

---

[9] Karl Marx, *Capital: A Critical Analysis of Capitalist Production*, Volume 1 (Moscow: Progress, 1965 [1867]), p. 35.

[10] Marx, *Capital*, p. 36.

become more and more abstracted from the material that designates it (the actual paper dollar or metal coins standing for parts of a dollar like quarters or cents). The price is an exchange value articulated in a monetary quantity. Commodities that are quite different from each other have the same price (an Atkins cookbook costs as much as an Atkins container of supplements and several food products) so from the perspective of money there are no qualitative differences whatsoever. Everything is the same. Everything has only exchange-value.

The perspective of money is also the perspective of the capitalists, the people who have capital (hence the money) to invest in factory buildings, machinery, raw materials, and a labor force, all the necessary pieces for the production of something for a capitalist market. The perspective of the capitalists is, then, that of exchange-value. The capitalists are not interested in use-values since for them investments of their capital are a means for the accumulation of further capital and increased capitalization does not take place without an exchange that yields the best of exchange-values, more money. "Use values are only produced by the capitalists because and in so far as, they are the material substratum, the depositories of exchange-value,"[11] states Marx.

If it is indeed the case that capitalists produce use-values only insofar as utility is needed in order for something to have an exchange value, then from the perspective of the capitalists it is not accommodation that motivates the production of commodities (since after all what they are after is an exchange). Yet, it is important for the capitalists that commodities be perceived as accommodating whether they actually are or not (in view of the fact that otherwise there will be no exchange and the items they try to sell will not be sold). Capitalists, therefore have a vested interest in consumers taking surface appearances as reality, in a lack of distinction between appearance and reality, and in the creation of the most solid possible impression that the products that their enterprises put on the market are indeed real commodities. To a great extent this is what advertisement is all about.

Since people have needs, what they have to be convinced of is that some product can indeed satisfy them (it has the use-value

---

[11] Marx, *Capital*, p. 186.

they seek) and do it better than competing products (and is, therefore, the commodity they want). People, of course, can also have wants that are not need based and wants that may not even mesh with any needs. Indeed people can have wants that are manufactured by the advertisements for specific products. Advertisment-based wants include, for example, many of the wants of children who are bombarded with advertisements for unnecessary products while watching children's TV shows. People need to eat and drink. It's better for people to be healthy. It's impossible for people to be young forever. Is the Atkins Diet a commodity or is it a simulation or a conjured-up imitation of a commodity?

Alienating Diets

To the extent that advertising works it is not due to how clever advertisers are and how stupid the rest of us are in comparison. At least, Marx would have not thought so. Marx would have correlated the success of advertising with a phenomenon he called alienation. For Marx, alienation is a social phenomenon—not the individual psychological feeling of not belonging, which is a psychological phenomenon. Because it is a social rather than a psychological phenomenon, while one necessarily experiences alienation, one may, nonetheless, not feel alienated. Alienation begins with the "estrangement of labor." Labor is always externalized in some fashion, in writing, for example, cooking, or in building. Labor can become estranged when in addition to its externalization it also becomes separated from the laborer, the person who labors in writing, cooking, or building. Labor becomes separated from the laborer in a unique kind of way when it is sold, which is what one does when placing oneself on a labor market in order to get a job. Once separated (sold), it does not belong to the laborer anymore and worse, it becomes foreign and unfamiliar, hence, fully alien. This does not happen whenever one works (since work can take place without the selling of labor) but rather when work takes place within the capitalist system and becomes a commodity.

The capitalist system is a social formation that can be characterized in many ways. In order to understand alienation, what one needs to realize is that it divides people into classes. Of these, one is the capitalist class, which owns so much of the available capital that it has control over it.[12] The other classes stand in some relation to the capitalist class. Due to the capitalist control of capital, the members of these other classes are dependent on the capitalists for their livelihood. Capitalist control of capital turns capitalists into the source of all jobs, be these highly paid like those of corporate lawyers or badly paid like those of janitors. Dependence for work, without which one cannot enter the market as a consumer of the commodities one needs and wants in one's life, reveals an element of un-freedom in work. One can experience this un-freedom as one shapes and reshapes one's work life to fit the market, denying rather than affirming oneself as one does so. One studies medicine though one wants to be an artist, for example, or having studied to be a photographer one retrains and becomes a web designer. Whenever, one does this, an internal split takes place, and in addition, that part of oneself that one shapes for work becomes external in the process of looking for a job since jobs themselves are in a market in which the working part of the self is a commodity that has an exchange-value if it has a marketable use-value.[13] Capitalist job markets are, after all, just another kind of capitalist commodity markets. Another route to getting at the experience of alienation requires a return to the analysis of commodities as products produced for a market to be exchanged, including labor power (a person's job skills) in the set of all commodities. In markets, everything and everyone stand to everything and everyone in an exchange relationship. Everything and everyone is exchangeable for everything and everyone else. Networks of exchange are all there is, not only with respect to the relations among things, but also to all social relations.[14]

One is alienated due to one's lack of freedom. This is an alienation from oneself. One is also alienated from others and this is due to thoroughgoing commodification, the placement of

---

[12] For an example see http://faireconomy.org/research/wealth_charts.html (accessed March 2005). The charts at this site call attention to the distribution of wealth in the United States.

[13] For Marx's analysis of alienation, see "Economic and Philosophic Manuscripts of 1844" in *Karl Marx and Frederick Engels Collected Works*, Volume 3 (New York: International, 1975), especially pp. 270–283.

[14] See Marx's analysis of the fetishism of commodities, *Capital*, pp. 71–83.

everything in an exchange nexus. The two mutually reinforce each other because humans are fundamentally social. People become even more alien to themselves due to their alienation from each other and they necessarily become more alien to each other the more alien they are to themselves. In conditions of such deep and criss-crossing alienation one cannot easily exercise critical reflective judgment since it requires a connecting with others on a plane other than an exchange plane. But, the exchange plane is very hard to escape and in a way that will facilitate critical reflective judgment rather than intimacy, romanticism, and nostalgia. This is why advertising works. It does not manipulate. It represents our reality to us by representing us in exchange relations. It thus also constructs our reality and us since it places us in both familiar and less familiar exchange relations as it tries to represent the totality of possible exchange relations.

Advertising can be more or less sophisticated in its representations. The advertising for the Atkins Diet is quite sophisticated. It positions one first and foremost in relation to oneself seemingly giving one control over one's life (which one may want to grab to compensate for one's lack of freedom). At the same time it mediates the individual relationship to one's self by refereeing and configuring one's relationship to food and drink, two of the basics of sheer survival. It thereby infantilizes one quite immediately since the Atkins Diet is now in the place of a parent who knows better than the child what the child should eat. To take that place more firmly, it offers not only information about the diet and fitting recipes (a commodity with exchange value), but also food and drink products and dietary supplements (commodities with exchange-value) ready made for consumption. In the final analysis, then, the relationship of oneself to oneself is mediated via exchange. Because this relationship is also rather isolated from a relationship to others (the website does not even have a forum to simulate community in virtual space), it is even more striking how much the relationship with the self that the Atkins Diet offers is mediated via exchange.

Why Not the Atkins Diet?

Having said all of the above, I realize that I am not going to convince anyone not to go "on" the Atkins Diet. All diets seem to be alike if they are diets one is to try, especially in order to lose weight. Moreover the Atkins Diet can be quite sumptuous as indicated by the pictures of the permissible foods. So why not the Atkins Diet?

Perhaps because it is luxurious.

I am not saying this because I am against eating well or against eating good food. I do think, however, that low-carb diets rely on the consumption of meats of all sorts since they are the best and easiest source of protein. The majority of the world eats high-carb diets and does so because it is poor, not because it prefers high-carb foods. The poorest of the people in the world—those who are truly without food—do not need to go on weight-loss diets, though due to globalization and changes in the available foods for poor people globally, many poor people worldwide are actually obese.

So there's something paradoxical in a weight-loss diet such as the Atkins Diet, intended for people who have more means than most and offering them a weight loss that does not require a re-evaluation of the means at their disposal. A diet aimed only at the privileged testifies further to the kind of alienation of which Marx speaks.

11

Bias and Body Size: The Social Contract and the Fat Liberation Movement

ABBY WILKERSON

Imagine a world in which you, as a fat person, are likely to be regarded by prospective employers as less reliable than others, or not the right image to represent the organization.[1] No matter how healthy you are, you have trouble getting access to affordable health insurance. You delay seeing a doctor because of unpleasant past experiences, but when you do visit one, with an upper respiratory infection you can't get rid of, you are weighed in full view of everyone in the hallway, and given a gown that doesn't cover you. Your doctor then discusses weight loss with you rather than the symptoms that brought you there. When you attend a concert or movie, or travel for vacation or work, the seats do not accommodate you because "normal" size has been defined as smaller than you—and you may even be required to pay for two seats so that others are not crowded. Relaxing at home, you turn on the TV to hear antifat jokes on one channel and weight-loss talk on the next. In short, you face an array of difficulties getting through each day, because of how that social world has been arranged.

This, of course, is the world we now inhabit. It's hard to overstate the influence of the slenderness norm, yet it does face opposition. The Fat Liberation movement demands recognition

[1] The author wishes to thank the editors of this volume as well as Cynthia Newcomer for their thoughtful commentary which greatly improved this essay. Furthermore, Lisa Heldke first suggested the provocative connection between the Fat Liberation Movement and social contract theory.

of fatness as ordinary human variation rather than medical pathology or flaw in character or appearance. Another world, they say, is possible.[2] Imagine a world without fat jokes, carb counting, mandatory weigh-ins, endless self-monitoring for weight and body shape. Imagine a world in which our bodies and minds are free of this self-scrutiny, a world in which dignity comes in all shapes and sizes. Imagine a world in which others listen to what fat people have to say, fat people who speak with authority about their own bodies and lives without apology or any promise to lose weight.

The Atkins program offers to help fat people overcome the condition that singles them out—but Fat Liberationists respond that the condition that needs to be corrected is social intolerance, not fatness. In their view, the problem is not obesity but systematic discrimination: a breach of the social contract, a systematic devaluation of an entire group, on the basis of widely held, if faulty, medical evidence. Undoubtedly the most influential value underlying both the rationale for and the popularity of the Atkins Diet is the sense that it is bad to be fat, and the Fat Liberation movement has shown that, as a social response to fatness, this value is indeed political in nature. Fat Liberation activists view the expectation that fat people must diet as a form of oppression.

Atkins Diet literature also views fatness as a social issue, concentrating intensively on the interactions of fat people with others. Given that both sides of this divide frame the debate in these overtly social and political terms, the Atkins Diet, considered as a social response to fatness, is a provocative topic for political philosophy, and for social contract theory in particular. Atkins claims that it is the only diet plan to provide dramatic results that last, to promote health and safety, and to give satisfying food options that keep dieters from feeling deprived—yet evidence indicates that none of these claims holds up. Its persistence and popularity need an explanation. Understanding it as a political phenomenon—particularly how it both reflects and

---

[2] I am appropriating "Another world is possible," the slogan made famous at the Seattle Protest of the antiglobalization movement. I extend it to the context of obesity, which has received little critical attention within this movement, but in my view is inextricably connected with the movement's concern with the impact of corporate practices on individual health and food security.

reinforces the individualism of our culture—can help provide one.

Following the lead of Fat Liberationists, I use "fat" as a neutral descriptive term, in contrast to its pejorative connotation in standard usage. In a piece called "Why I Encourage You to Use the F-Word," activist and author Marilyn Wann contends that "fat" is "the least offensive, simplest word on the subject"—in contrast to terms like "obese" and "overweight" that reflect medical assumptions that are questionable at best, or euphemisms such as "heavy, large, voluptuous, zaftig, big-boned," intended to politely conceal a "distasteful" reality.[3] In short, Wann says, "There is nothing wrong with being fat, so there's nothing wrong with using the word" (FS, p. 20).

Fatness and the Social Contract

What justifies the existence of the state—why should individuals accept the constraints on their autonomy that the state requires? Philosophers have responded to this question using the social contract, an imaginary construct that founds the mutual obligations between citizens and the state. Thomas Hobbes, for example, argued in 1651 that rationality and self-interest are the basis of morality and the shared governance of society. While men, in his view, are by nature selfish, rationality makes it clear that mutual restraint of self-interest brings about the mutual advantages that shared governance can provide, and thus the basis for the social contract is secure.[4]

There are many versions of social contract theory, including versions that take into account information about specific social conditions. Recently, some theorists have used social contract theory to examine the relationship of marginalized groups to

---

[3] Marilyn Wann, *Fat! So? Because You Don't Have to Apologize for Your Size* (Berkeley: Ten Speed Press, 1998), pp. 19, 20. Hereafter referred to in text as FS.

[4] Thomas Hobbes, *Leviathan* (Harmondsworth: Penguin, 1985). I use the gender-specific term "men" intentionally here. Some philosophers say we should understand "men" in this context to refer to human beings in general. A number of feminist critics, however, argue persuasively that it should be understood in the literal, gender-specific sense in which it was clearly intended at the time, and that the sexism and patriarchy of Hobbes's time influence his theory in ways that prevent it from working in gender-neutral ways.

mainstream society. Following their lead, I will apply some key concepts from social contract theory to the politics of fatness, using the Atkins Diet to explore the social situation of fat people currently.

In recent years, anti-oppression theorists have looked to this social contract tradition as a means of critiquing existing social arrangements and envisioning more just alternatives. Carol Pateman argues that the social contract is synonymous with patriarchy and hence the oppression of women, and that historically and currently, the contract, functioning as a mode of agreement, has secured men's rights to control women's bodies through, for example, marriage, prostitution, and surrogate motherhood.[5] Charles Mills contends that a "racial contract" has been fundamental to the organization of Western society, and continues to structure it, defining full personhood and citizenship in ways that historically have excluded people of color, through a series of actual historical documents.[6] Both philosophers argue that social and political theory must attend carefully to current and ongoing social conditions, rather than continue the more abstract methodology that has prevailed.

One of the most original and significant aspects of their work is its challenge to the individualist paradigm of Western philosophy. Rather than focusing entirely on individuals and their relationship to the state, Pateman and Mills contend that we must look at society's treatment of particular groups in order to discover injustice and rectify it. They show that considering individuals in the abstract prevents us from recognizing injustice that occurs on the basis of social group membership. This insight of recent social contract theory can help us to reflect on the tensions between the profound individualism of dieting (which is more pronounced in the Atkins method than many) and the collective basis of fat oppression as well as liberation.

Antifat oppression is by no means the centuries-long tradition that racism, sexism, and heterosexism are in Western society. The relationship of fatness to the social contract is in this sense quite different from that of race or gender. Nonetheless, I contend that the slenderness norm and antifat bias have become

---

[5] Carol Pateman, *The Sexual Contract* (Stanford: Stanford University Press, 1988).

[6] Charles Mills, *The Racial Contract* (Ithaca: Cornell University Press, 1997).

a significant aspect of the current social contract, enforced in varying ways by most of the major institutions of society, including the family, education, medicine, employment, and mass media.[7] Weight loss and slenderness promotion of course play a major role in the economy, turning out significant profits for the pharmaceutical, surgical, fashion, publishing, popular diet, fitness, grocery, and, increasingly, restaurant industries, not to mention the marketing efforts that promote and sustain them all. Politics is nothing more and nothing less than the social distribution of power, which occurs through a range of cultural and economic forces in addition to formal legal rights and responsibilities. Antifat bias privileges some people (those who are not fat) at the expense of others (those who are). This form of oppression illustrates how groups can be systematically disadvantaged through cultural forces as well as through formal and legal policies and procedures.[8]

What role, then, does the Atkins Diet play in the sociopolitics of body size and shape? Its chief rationale, of course, is identical to that of other weight-loss methods: the dual aesthetic and medical goal of slimness and health. There's a moral element to this goal as well, since fatness is perceived as a failure of will or a lack of self-control. As perhaps the most prominent brand name associated with a diet plan, with an extensive website as well as many publications and a wide range of diet products, Atkins illustrates the profitability of diet marketing. Its phenomenal popularity as well as the strong criticism it has faced point to important social tensions regarding bodily control and the role of health in cultural definitions of personhood. While dieting itself is generally individualistic, especially as a social approach to significant public health problems, Atkins is much more individualist in its approach than plans such as Jenny Craig or Weight Watchers,[9] both of which

---

[7] Antifat norms seem less significant in religion than in other major social institutions. Nonetheless, a Google search for "'Christian weight loss'" turned up about 27,100 pages. (http://www.google.com/search?num=50&hl=en&lr=lang_en&q=%22christian+weight+loss%22&btnG=Search, accessed December 28, 2004).

[8] In my view, antifat bias also frequently serves to reinforce other modes of oppression, affecting many who are not considered fat, along with those who are (a point that space considerations do not allow me to develop here).

[9] I thank the Popular Culture and Philosophy series editor for this point.

include group participation and support components. The Atkins Diet claims to be (a) the most, indeed the only, safe and effective means of achieving weight loss, which in turn is (b) medically imperative in order to prevent catastrophic health consequences. Thus, the Atkins Diet positions itself as offering a helping hand to fat people—and implicitly as a private remedy for a punitive social environment.

Yet some fat people do not find the Atkins Diet helpful. Fat Liberation activists charge that such fat-related diagnoses as "morbid obesity" are grounded in conservative or discriminatory social ideology, that they mark a benign rather than pathological condition, and that the Atkins Diet is not only ineffective but potentially more harmful than the condition it is meant to treat. Fat activists understand their encounters with the institution of medicine as a human rights issue, in which medical authority functions to undermine their bodily integrity, self-determination, and basic self-regard. As they see it, insofar as the Atkins Diet justifies itself through standard medical notions of obesity, it is morally and scientifically problematic.

"Obesity" and Diets: Medical Considerations

Atkins for Life, the diet guru's guide to a long-term low-carb diet, begins by citing familiar concepts such as a recent increase in the weight of Americans, the deadliness of obesity, and its connection to many diseases.[10] After discussing these conditions and why he believes they are associated with "excessive carbohydrate intake," (A, p. x) Atkins concludes: "Our approach to weight control is not just about looking slim—it is perhaps the most significant tool you have to influence your overall health and enhance your chances for a long and vigorous life" (A, p. x). He assures prospective dieters that "lab tests showing their changed blood sugar, cholesterol, and triglyceride levels will be tangible evidence of that improvement" in health (A, p. xi). Atkins's skillful use of this medical discourse of obesity is clearly a key factor in the program's success. Within this discourse, health is conceived as a property of individuals, an idea which

---

[10] Robert C. Atkins, M.D., *Atkins for Life* (New York: St. Martin's, 2003), pp. ix–xi. Hereafter referred to in text as A.

might seem unremarkable at first, but which has faced significant challenges that I will return to shortly.

Significant challenges have been raised to both the general claims about the poor-health consequences of "obesity" and the specific claims about the merits of the Atkins program as a means for correcting or preventing these problems. The prevailing medical discourse about fatness also reflects and sustains social prejudices against fatness. Moreover, the ideologically determined concept of "obesity" represents the willful expert ignorance of everyone's real body,[11] in particular the oft-cited majority of people in the United States now considered to be "overweight" based on Body Mass Index.[12]

A significant body of medical evidence indicates it is quite possible to be both fat and healthy. A Cooper Fitness Institute study found that physically active fat people had higher levels of cardiovascular fitness (as measured by treadmill stress tests) than inactive thin people.[13] A growing number of researchers defend the viability of "Health at Every Size," concluding that it is physical activity and healthy eating (that is, eating a variety of nutritious foods) rather than weight that influence health.[14] Correlations between fatness and poor health have been demonstrated, but the *causal* power of fatness has not, while there is positive evidence of other factors (including dieting itself) as the determining factors in the poor health conditions that have been linked with fatness. The notion of obesity as epidemic presupposes individual responsibility for health and well-being, and perceives the body as both a reflection of individual character and a metaphor for the moral, political, and economic state of society—failing to acknowledge the considerable environmental influences on health status.

---

[11] See Susan Wendell, "Toward a Feminist Theory of Disability," in Lennard Davis, ed., *The Disability Studies Reader* (New York: Routledge, 1997), p. 267.

[12] Blogger Paul McAleer lampoons the arbitrariness of "the Night You Became Fat (that is, when the BMI changed literally overnight)," resulting in an instant rise in American overweight statistics. "Obesity Statistics Seriously Flawed," *Big Fat Blog*, 24th October, 2003: http://www.bigfatblog.com/archives/001069.php (accessed 28th December, 2004).

[13] Boston Women's Health Book Collective, *Our Bodies, Ourselves for the New Century* (New York: Touchstone, 1998), p. 60.

[14] See Paul Campos, *The Obesity Myth* (New York: Gotham, 2004), pp. 173–181.

Research indicates that people of color are more likely than Caucasians both to be fat and to face certain health risks; low socioeconomic status also increases the likelihood of both, due to diet along with many other reasons.[15] The food accessible and affordable to poor people is usually highly processed, based on refined starches, and high in the unhealthiest fats, making a nutritious diet very difficult for poor people to achieve. Instead of grocery stores, the poorest areas of many cities have only fast-food outlets and convenience stores that do not sell fresh produce, nor are there safe parks or other areas that encourage physical activity. Social and economic disparities such as these influence *both* fatness and poor health, rather than fatness being the cart that drives the horse.

Trans-fatty acids and high-fructose corn syrup (or HFCS), found in virtually all processed and fast foods, directly undermine health. Trans-fatty acids (oils that have been partially hydrogenated to transform them into shelf-stable solid shortening) are banned in Europe as a leading cause of high cholesterol (a well-verified health risk), yet pervasive in the U.S. diet.[16] HFCS is associated with liver dysfunction and coronary disease and contributes to elevated blood triglycerides in men; it is metabolized differently than other sugars, processed more like a fat than a sugar.[17] A number of researchers have identified the rise in HFCS consumption as an important factor in the increase in diabetes rates.[18] In 2001, people in the U.S. consumed an average of 62.5 pounds each of HFCS in sodas, baked goods, and other products;[19] an estimated 10 percent of all calories con-

---

[15] *National Heart, Lung, and Blood Institute of the National Institutes of Health*, "Guidelines on Overweight and Obesity," http://nhlbi.nih.gov/guidelines/obesity/e_txtbk/intro/intro.htm (accessed 17th March, 2004).

[16] *Our Bodies, Ourselves*, p. 49.

[17] Sally Squires, "Sweet but Not So Innocent? High-Fructose Corn Syrup May Act More Like Fat Than Sugar in the Body," *Washington Post* (11th March, 2003): http://www.washingtonpost.com/ac2/wp-dyn/A8003-2003Mar10?language=printerwashingtonpost.com (accessed 17th March, 2003).

[18] Michael Pollan, "Industrial Corn—Destroying Our Health & Environment: When a Crop Becomes King," *New York Times* (18th July, 2002), reprinted in *Organic Consumers Association*, http://www.organicconsumers.org/toxic/toomuchcorn071902.cfm (accessed 17th March, 2003); Squires, "Sweet but Not So Innocent?"

[19] Squires, "Sweet but Not So Innocent?"

sumed in the U.S. now come from HFCS, with many children getting 20 percent of their calories from it.[20] Many of the problems associated with fatness are very likely related to consumption of these ingredients, which take considerable effort to avoid, rather than to weight itself.

The social status of fat people directly harms their health. Social stigmas against fatness are another important environmental factor strongly influencing the health of fat people. The extreme stress linked to stigma, prejudice, and discrimination (as with other forms of oppression, particularly those based on visible characteristics) has an array of negative health consequences, including high blood pressure, depression, digestive problems, headaches, and other chronic illnesses (FS, p. 36). Stigmas against fatness can discourage fat people's fitness efforts when they are singled out and harassed at health clubs, swimming pools, jogging trails, and other public sites, provoking feelings of exposure, shame, and vulnerability. Physicians' attitudes to fatness impose obstacles to health care as well; fat people repeatedly attest to being treated for weight itself rather than for acute illnesses that brought them to the doctor in the first place. Betty Rose Dudley's doctor, for example, insisted on discussing weight loss techniques with her rather than a lung abnormality that could be cancer (FS, pp. 42–43).

Another health risk imposed on fat people is dieting itself, a particularly disturbing risk given the association between dieting and health. Diets generally fall below the level of caloric intake identified as starvation by the World Health Organization.[21] Dieting, especially repeatedly, can lead to depression, tissue damage, slowed metabolism, altered sense of satiety, uncontrollable craving, regained weight (often in the form of increased abdominal fat, with its higher risk of heart disease), and loss of muscle tissue, often replaced by body fat.[22] Atkins claims that its high-protein, low-carb, unrestricted fat approach is what makes it uniquely effective for health and weight loss and superior to calorie counting, yet a comparative study of several popular diets over a year suggests that any effectiveness of the Atkins

---

[20] Pollan, "Industrial Corn."

[21] *Our Bodies, Ourselves*, p. 59.

[22] *Ibid.*, p. 59.

program ultimately rests on the calorie restriction that turns out to be an effect, if not the goal, of its methods. Moreover, Atkins came in last in effectiveness of all the diets studied.[23]

To review the overall implications of this discussion for Atkins specifically, let us consider what is unique to Atkins as a diet program. It's not the only low-carbohydrate diet, but it certainly goes further than others in reducing carbohydrate intake while increasing protein and allowing a fairly high proportion of fat, and thus, unlike some diets, is palatable to people who enjoy eating meat and feel deprived by limiting fats. The health benefits of reducing or eliminating consumption of refined carbohydrates, one of the key principles of the diet, are clear, given the role of refined carbohydrate consumption in developing diabetes. Those who follow this principle will eliminate high-fructose corn syrup from their diets, of course, and thereby avoid its known risks to health. There is also some merit to Atkins's critique of low-fat diets, insofar as they avoid beneficial fats along with harmful ones, and foods typically consumed on these diets, especially commercially available low-fat products, often are laden with refined sweeteners to compensate for the fat that has been removed. To their credit, recent Atkins publications also warn readers of the dangers of trans fats.

Yet there is growing evidence (some of which I have already noted) that the health and efficacy advantages claimed by the Atkins Diet cannot be supported. First of all, as many critics have pointed out, Atkins eliminates beneficial unrefined carbohydrates found in unprocessed grains, fruits, and vegetables in the early phase of the diet, and continues to restrict their consumption significantly in the intermediate and ongoing phases, depriving the diet of necessary fiber and a range of nutrients. A range of health problems are associated with the program—due not only to carb restriction but also to the emphasis on foods tending to be high in cholesterol and unhealthy fats.

---

[23] M.L. Dansinger, J.L. Gleason, J.L. Griffith., *et al.*, "One Year Effectiveness of the Atkins, Ornish, Weight Watchers, and Zone Diets in Decreasing Body Weight and Heart Disease Risk," presented at the American Heart Association Scientific Sessions (12th November, 2003) in Orlando. Cited in "Atkins Nutritional Approach," in *Wikipedia: The Free Encyclopedia*: http://en.wikipedia.org/wiki/Atkins_Nutritional_Approach (accessed 28th December, 2004).

At a deeper level, because it is grounded in the individualist discourse of medicine, the Atkins program chooses to target individuals rather than to challenge the corporate interests perpetuating the health problems that it supposedly tries to prevent—and it actually profits from environmentally caused health problems by constituting itself as a consumer choice available in the marketplace for those who can afford to pursue it as a means, however illusory, of seeking health. It also contributes to the public confusion that results from conflating the benign characteristic of weight with health problems such as heart disease and diabetes. Despite a wealth of information documenting these serious flaws of the Atkins program, it continues to position itself as a marketplace competitor to other diets rather than to challenge directly the environmental problems and political interests that undermine the health of individuals. In doing so, it is one of the most prominent promoters of society's antifat imperative, and thus a major contributor to a social contract that is disempowering to fat people. It also contributes significantly to this disempowerment by recasting deeply social problems as the responsibility of the individuals who bear the brunt of them—and maintains its own stake in those problems never being perceived as political in nature, let alone addressed as such.

The Social World of Atkins

Atkins for Life is filled with individual stories that intertwine significant weight loss with dramatic social and interpersonal victories. The main text of each chapter is in the voice of Dr. Atkins, occasionally incorporating brief individual stories in the third person. Longer first-person stories appear between chapters, complete with before and after photos and sidebars with personal statistics as well as each individual's weight loss tips. While health is a core value addressed in every story, weight loss as a means of connecting with others also plays a major role. Taken together, these stories present a compelling portrait of the social situation of fat people, which the diet seems intended to rectify along with excess weight. Since the Atkins plan is meant to be followed on one's own rather than through structured group activities, it is a more individualistic version of what is already a highly individual cultural pursuit, since every diet requires constant and intensive self-monitoring. This individualism, as noted before, functions to obscure oppressive aspects of the social contract, recasting them as individual failings. At the same time, however, the personal narratives suggest that others will rally to support one's efforts, and, even more importantly, that following the program will integrate one more fully and satisfyingly into society and may even resolve interpersonal challenges—implicit testimony to the significance of group status, the central concern of the social contract theorists identified above.

Atkins presents the value of weight loss in ways that assume the merits of traditional gender roles—the very assumption challenged by social contract theorists concerned with gender justice. When women discuss fitness, their stories tend to frame physical activity in terms of relationships with others. Exercise is not only a means of weight loss and health promotion, but also a way to interact with others that was out of reach before participating in Atkins, and even a way of permanently establishing new ties. Kerry Feather, for example, had missed the athleticism she enjoyed before gaining weight. Once she lost sixty pounds, she says, "I started to get my volleyball game back. I also began dating the man who became my new husband. He was a fellow teammate and together we started running" (A, p. 99). Women dieters with children also tend to link fitness with their roles as mothers. After losing seventy-five pounds, Luann Lockhart says, "I have enough energy to referee volleyball and keep up with my seventeen-year-old daughter" (A, p. 22). April Greer reports that as a result of her ninety-nine-pound loss, "Now, instead of sitting on the couch watching television, I play football with my sons, who are nine and six" (p. 29). These new opportunities in relationships serve as a means of integration into society in traditional ways, not only strengthening the women's ties with others but bolstering their social roles as wives and mothers.

On the surface, the stories are very upbeat, emphasizing health, energy, newfound career success, and an overall renewed enthusiasm for living. Yet a past of loneliness, shame, and isolation—exclusion from the social contract—is repeatedly evoked as the background contrast to this present-day foreground of health and zest. Luann Lockhart, the woman who lost seventy-five pounds, says, "People look at me differently [. . .]. Even though my daughter never said anything about it, I could tell that having a heavy mother embarrassed her. Now she's proud of me. In fact, when we go out together, people think we're sisters!" (A, p. 23). Matthew Holloway says that as a result of his weight loss, "I went swimming recently and took off my shirt in public for the first time in thirteen years. My social life is better than I ever dreamed. [. . .] Doing Atkins saved my life and changed me completely" (A, p. 31). Terry Free says of life after weight loss, "I don't get depressed by wondering if people are thinking, 'Gee, that guy is fat!'"(A, p. 84). Ralph Drake weighed 280 pounds (much of which he had regained after an earlier bout with Atkins) and lost over 100; now, "Newly married and with twin babies, Ralph has everything to live for"—suggesting that those who are fat, unmarried, and childless must be living lives that are lonely, meaningless, and unhappy, all because of fatness (A, p. 22).

Christianne Bishop's concern with appearance reflects its centrality in a number of stories. Around her fiftieth birthday, Bishop writes, "I had long, brown hair and 'Coke-bottle' glasses. . . . my weight had gradually crept up to 160. I felt like a fat blob"(A, p. 65). By January, a few weeks later, "I was down to 134 pounds. By mid-June, I weighed only 115 pounds and stopped keeping records. I cut my hair and dyed it blond and also had Lasik surgery to correct my eyesight" (A, p. 66). Bishop concludes her section with an inspiring thought: "Our strength comes from within, and there is truly no limit to what we can do"—yet readers are left with the distinct impression that no amount of inner strength can compensate for an exterior that others consider unattractive (A, p. 66). Stories like these contribute to a social climate of harsh standards for personal appearance, and increasing pressures to find consumer solutions to such "problems" rather than to confront the standards themselves as unjust.

If the values that motivate weight loss, the many negative associations of fatness, come from the larger social context, the motivation to continue the struggle also frequently has important collective elements. Not only is the end result of weight loss associated with newfound connections to others, the very *effort* to lose weight via Atkins methods is also depicted as a means of connecting. The stories obscure the need to challenge an oppressive social contract by showing people integrating themselves into society by dieting, which seems to serve as their public affirmation of social norms. In many stories, beginning the Atkins programs provides an opportunity for the dieter's partner, friends, families, or coworkers to connect in new ways with the dieter through helping with the project. Terry Free took up the Atkins Diet as a friendly competition with three other men, met his first goal, and decided to set another, timed for an extended family gathering for a cousin's graduation. Reaching that goal, he moved his mother to tears with his success, and got the attention of many others: "By this time, a day didn't go by that someone didn't ask me how I'd lost the weight. I had become a phenomenon. It was such a hoot and a holler when people didn't recognize me. . . . people in the office began to bring me clothes that no longer fit them or their family members" (A, p. 83). He became a "coach" to co-workers impressed with his results.

Behind these stories conveying the inspirational value of others' support in weight loss lurks the distinct suspicion that you can never really be part of the group in the same way if you are fat and not doing anything about it. While Atkins's book restricts the rationale for weight loss mainly to health, the stories told by the dieters cite the value of transformed interactions with others with such regularity that it becomes the main subtext of their stories. The message that a mother should alter her own body to deal with her daughter's embarrassment about it, and that there is no higher compliment than that you look younger than you are, conveys the conditional character of social acceptance very clearly. The need to cover one's body in public, even while swimming, is just one of the many examples of internalized shame over others' perceptions of one's body that come up in almost every story, eloquently attesting to the link between social rejection and fatness or weight gain. Considering that the stories encompass the domains of work, education, friendship, athletics, and both romantic and family relationships, a clear picture emerges that there is no place to escape from antifat stigma and the exclusion and isolation that result. This is clear and powerful testimony to how these institutions work together systematically to enforce a social contract disempowering to fat people. Dieting seems to have become a kind of ritual self-abasement, a preemptive public admission of one's own inadequacy that has been learned through social interaction. In this sense the admission implied by dieting is what is required, gaining social approval like that of weight loss itself. Perhaps this helps explain the persistence of diets and recommendations to follow them despite the strong evidence that they are neither safe nor effective.

Another World Is Possible: The Social World of Fat Liberation

Even though Fat Liberationists may not use the philosophical language of the social contract, I hope to have shown that their position is congruent with an understanding of society's antifat attitudes as a breach of the social contract, rationalized through faulty medical evidence. "But what about health?," many readers will be unable to avoid asking in response. Indeed, many of us need to be more active, to eat better food and eliminate the worst foods from our diets, and to watch cholesterol and blood sugar levels.[24] Yet these goals are just as vital for thin people as for fat ones, so it makes no sense to single out fat people with this message. Moreover, these goals are far more attainable than the medical and social imperative to lose weight, and so should replace the latter entirely. Doing so promotes public health far more effectively, especially considering that heart disease and diabetes, the afflictions most often associated with fatness, certainly affect thin people as well as those who are not, and their needs should not be overlooked. It also is far more consistent with the democratic values that mandate respect for all members of society.

The Atkins program offers to help fat people overcome the condition that singles them out. Fat Liberationists respond that the condition that needs to be corrected is social intolerance, not fatness. Imagine a world in which anyone can work out or eat or dress flamboyantly in public without being harassed—or visit the doctor with a pressing concern without being lectured about self-control. Imagine a world in which no one is automatically discounted because of their appearance when they speak about their own body or health. Imagine a world in which everyone has the option and the means to choose healthy foods and to enjoy being physically active. What if the considerable resources

---

[24] See Wann, *Fat! So?* especially pp. 35–41, 56–62, and 87–88.

of the Atkins enterprise, indeed all the social resources devoted to promoting antifat bias, were instead diverted to these goals? Efforts in this direction will benefit not only fat people but other oppressed groups as well. Another world is possible.

12
A Vegetarian's Beef with Atkins

DAVID DETMER

All fruits, vegetables, and grains contain carbohydrates. Meats, on the other hand, while often high in fat content, generally are very low in carbohydrates. Consequently, the Atkins Diet, which emphasizes high-protein, low-carbohydrate foods while permitting the consumption of high-fat foods, presents itself as a weight-conscious meat-lover's dream. Indeed, the late Dr. Atkins himself pointed out that many people who take up his diet do so in part because he "certainly won't discourage them from eating meat, fish and fowl." He could not have done so without hypocrisy, since he was, as he cheerfully admitted, "a carnivore, too."[1]

But should we be carnivores? Is there anything morally objectionable about the practice of eating animal flesh?

Traditional (or "commonsense") morality would seem to answer that there is nothing wrong with eating meat. The vast majority of people in the United States and in other Western industrialized nations do so, often without giving the matter a second thought. While they may be aware that some vegetarians reject the practice of meat eating for moral reasons, they are

[1] Robert C. Atkins, M.D., *Dr. Atkins' New Diet Revolution* (New York: Avon, 2002), p. 90. Atkins explicitly acknowledges that his diet is not vegetarian-friendly. He notes that strict vegetarians "really can't do the Induction phase," and that those who avoid red meat will have difficulty sticking to the later phases if they do not at least eat fish, chicken, eggs, and cheese (*New Diet Revolution*, 149).

likely to think that such a minority position must rest on some conception of morality that differs radically from their own.

But I will argue that "moral vegetarianism"—the doctrine that vegetarianism is morally obligatory, and the consumption of meat immoral (at least for those who, like most relatively wealthy North Americans and Europeans, have easy access to plant-based foods)—follows directly and logically from basic moral principles that nearly everyone already accepts.

The Wrongness of Cruelty

What are these "basic moral principles"? One is simply that cruelty—the infliction of unnecessary suffering on others—is morally wrong. Let's look at an example. Suppose my dentist causes me to suffer. Under what circumstances should we regard his conduct as wrong?[2] Well, suppose that the entire point of his actions is to hurt me. He is a sadist who enjoys causing others to suffer. We should condemn his actions as cruel and, for that reason, wrong. To vary the example, let's next imagine that, while the actions through which he hurts me benefit me significantly (they improve the health of my teeth and gums) and are undertaken for that reason, he could have benefited me in exactly the same way without hurting me (he was too lazy, or indifferent to my suffering, to bother with using an anesthetic). This, too, is cruel, but for a different reason. The infliction of pain was in a sense unintentional (it wasn't desired for its own sake), but the suffering was unnecessary and easily preventable, and it was not prevented only because of a moral failing (laziness or indifference to the suffering of others). Lastly, suppose that while the pain is inflicted in order to bring about some benefit, and that the pain is necessary in order to bring about that benefit, the benefit derived is rather trivial, and certainly is not of sufficient magnitude as to warrant my undergoing the suffering. To cause others to suffer greatly in order to bring about insignificant benefits is also cruel and, for that reason, wrong. Thus, in order for the infliction of suffering on others to be morally justifiable, it would seem to have to pass two tests, which might be labeled the

[2] I use the masculine adjective only because my dentist is, in fact, male.

"necessity" test and the "proportion" test. To inflict suffering that isn't necessary (either as cause or consequence)[3] to the bringing about of some good isn't justifiable. Neither is the infliction of suffering that is disproportionately large in comparison to the small benefit to be derived from the infliction of the suffering.[4]

Vegetarianism

What has any of this to do with vegetarianism? Well, let's begin by noticing that even though most people hold that humans are of vastly greater moral worth than other animals, they also tend to think that cruelty to animals is wrong. And they seem to mean by this not only that it is wrong to torture animals for fun, but also that it is wrong to inflict significant pain on them for trivial or ignoble reasons, or to cause them pain that could easily be prevented, or to hurt them in order to attain goods that could easily be attained through other, painless, means.

What sorts of actions are condemned by this principle? Consider

> the treatment of the civet cat, a highly intelligent and sociable animal. Civet cats are trapped and placed in small cages inside darkened sheds, where fires keep the temperature up to 110º Fahrenheit. They are confined in this way until they die. What justifies this extraordinary mistreatment? These animals have the misfortune to produce a substance that is useful in the manufacture of perfume. Musk, which is scraped from their genitals once a day for as long as they can survive, makes the scent of perfume last a bit longer after each application. (The heat increases their "production" of musk.)[5]

---

[3] If I hire one candidate for a job over another, the one who does not get the job may well suffer as a result. But if I have only one job to give away (and let us suppose that it is an important job—one that will greatly benefit the community), this suffering is a necessary consequence of the hiring process.

[4] I don't mean to suggest that these two tests are the only relevant ones. For example, there is also the very important issue of the victim's consent, or lack thereof, to receive pain.

[5] James Rachels, "The Moral Argument for Vegetarianism," in Steven M. Cahn, ed., *Philosophy for the Twenty-First Century* (New York: Oxford University Press, 2003), p. 691.

I've been presenting this example to students for years. I find that nearly all of them are quick to condemn this treatment of civet cats, and, without prompting from me, to offer as their explanation that satisfactory perfumes can probably be made from synthetic or plant-based materials, and that, in any case, perfume isn't a sufficiently important good as to justify such an infliction of pain on animals. Many of them, eager to try to block the argument from moving in the direction of supporting vegetarianism, are then equally quick to contrast the case of civet cats with that of livestock. Cows, pigs, and chickens, they claim, are treated better than are the civet cats. And while perfume is a trivial luxury, meat, they confidently assert, is a vital necessity.

But these claims are simply untrue. Animals on modern factory farms are routinely, and not just occasionally, subjected to treatment far more horrific than that to which the unfortunate civet cats are subjected.[6] I will offer just one example.

> Nearly all beef producers . . . castrate their animals. . . . Castration is practiced because steers are thought to put on weight better than bulls . . . and because of a fear that the male hormones will cause a taint to develop in the flesh. Castrated animals are also easier to handle. Most farmers admit that the operation causes shock and pain to the animal. Anesthetics are generally not used. The procedure is to pin the animal down, take a knife, and slit the scrotum, exposing the testicles. You then grab each testicle in turn and pull on it, breaking the cord that attaches it; on older animals it may be necessary to cut the cord.[7]

Perhaps such treatment would be justified if it were the case that meat consumption is necessary for human health. But it isn't. We can nourish ourselves quite well without eating animals. Consequently, it appears that the justification for the massive pain that is inflicted on meat animals is simply that we like the taste of meat (or, perhaps, that we want a greater variety of tastes than we would have without eating meat). But these reasons seem rather trivial in comparison to the degree of suffering

---

[6] It would take many gruesome pages to document this claim adequately. The interested reader might begin by consulting Matthew Scully, *Dominion* (New York: St. Martin's, Griffin, 2002).

[7] Peter Singer, *Animal Liberation*, revised edition (New York: Avon, 1990), p. 145.

that the animals typically undergo. The analogy of the treatment of civet cats for perfume to the treatment of cows, pigs, and chickens for food therefore seems to hold. Both practices stand condemned as cruel, since they are instances of the infliction of significant suffering on others for the purpose of attaining rather trivial gains.

Is the Atkins Diet Cruel?

The significance of the Atkins Diet is that it offers another, less trivial, justification for eating meat. Perhaps by eating Dr. Atkins's heavily meat-oriented diet some people will be able to improve their health by losing weight. Since health is far from a trivial good, the infliction of suffering on factory farm animals for the purpose of enabling people to lose weight might then not count as cruel, according to the principles we've been considering.

To give this argument a fair chance, let's make several assumptions. First, let's make the assumption (which I find plausible), that obesity is generally, on balance, unhealthy, and that a moderately lean physique better lends itself to the enjoyment of good health. (Note that without this assumption the argument has little chance of succeeding, since the goal of satisfying one's vanity by looking good hardly seems sufficient to justify the horrific treatment to which meat animals are routinely subjected.) Let's assume, further, that the Atkins Diet is a uniquely effective one, and that, in particular, it offers the dieter a better chance of achieving optimum weight than does a well-planned vegetarian alternative.[8]

Even on these generous assumptions, it is far from clear that the Atkins Diet is morally defensible. After all, even on the most optimistic appraisal of the health benefits of weight loss, it might very well be doubted that the amount of good to be attained by the Atkins Diet is really proportionate to the degree of suffering

---

[8] I personally find this assumption quite dubious, and am making it here solely for the sake of argument. For a brief, informal, statement of some reasons for doubting the superior effectiveness of the Atkins Diet, see "The Diet War: Low-Fat vs. High-Protein with Dean Ornish," *WebMD*, at: http://my.webmd.com/content/article/53/60634.htm?lastselectedguid={5FE84E90-BC77-4056-A91C-9531713CA348} (accessed on 22nd February, 2005).

that must be inflicted on animals in order to facilitate it. And it is equally unclear that the Atkins Diet passes the necessity test. After all, even if one assumes that the Atkins Diet is the one that offers the best chance for successful weight loss, no one can reasonably claim that it is necessary to adopt the Atkins Diet in order to lose weight. Granted, it's difficult to reduce one's caloric intake while simultaneously increasing one's physical activity. Still, those who succeed in doing so over a long period of time usually achieve and maintain a desired weight loss. The advantage of the Atkins Diet, then, is that it makes weight control easier for some people by requiring less discipline of them. For example, it allows them to continue to eat some of the foods that they enjoy (namely, meat), that other diets might call for them to give up. But now we are back to trying to justify the massive infliction of animal suffering for the benefit of human convenience and taste, and that seems to run afoul of our scruples concerning cruelty to animals. Thus, the Atkins Diet appears to stand condemned on moral grounds.

The Moral Status of Human Beings

How might a defender of the Atkins Diet respond to this critique? The most likely move, I think, is to follow traditional morality in drawing an extremely sharp distinction between human beings and all other animals. Thus, even those defenders of the Atkins Diet who concede that it is wrong for one human being to inflict significant suffering on another human being unnecessarily, or for some relatively trivial purpose, might insist that such "cruelty" is justifiable if it is directed at animals. Such defenders might say that treatment of animals is objectionably cruel only if the pain that is inflicted on them is done for its own sake, as when it is done in pursuit of sadistic pleasure. But when it is done in pursuit of some otherwise unobjectionable human good, be it taste, vanity, entertainment, or what have you, it is justifiable. The reason is simply that humans "count" for more in moral reasoning than do other animals. We enjoy a significantly higher moral status.

But why is this so? On what grounds can one claim this exalted status for members of the human species? Why should we consider it to be morally acceptable to do to other animals what we would never do to humans? The natural and obvious response is to point out ways in which humans differ from other animals, and then to argue that these differences justify the differences in treatment. Accordingly, numerous thinkers have pointed to rationality, mastery of a language, the ability to reflect, and so on, as features a being must have in order to count substantially in moral deliberation, and as ones which, as luck would have it, humans, but no other animals, possess.[9]

In my judgment, this rationale for our current beliefs and practices is unsuccessful, since it cannot overcome two powerful and fundamental objections. The first is that there turns out to be no feature or set of features to which one can appeal to distinguish all humans from all nonhuman animals. Either one sets the bar high enough to exclude all nonhuman animals, in which case some humans—those who are severely retarded or brain-damaged, for example—will fail to make the cut, or else one sets the bar low enough to include all humans, in which case many animals will have to be included as well.

The other fundamental objection consists in questioning the moral relevance of the proposed feature or set of features. Consider, for example, the idea that what places human beings on a special moral plane is the fact that they, uniquely, can communicate in language. The obvious reply is that while this feature of human experience is morally relevant in some situations, it clearly is not in others. Thus, while the fact that a given pig can neither read nor write nor speak in a language provides an excellent reason to deny the pig admission to study in a university, it is far from clear how its linguistic capacities are relevant to the question of the moral legitimacy of causing the pig physical pain. Indeed, the utterance, "it's okay to hurt her—she can't talk," appears to be every bit as much a non sequitur as would "it's okay to hurt her—she's from Denver (or under six feet tall, or left-handed)." Thus, even if, contrary to fact, it were true that there are capacities shared by all humans but by no nonhuman animals, it wouldn't directly follow that this difference would justify any and every conceivable difference in treatment between people and animals. Rather, one would still have to show that the difference in question was relevant to the pro-

---

[9] See, for example, the selections by Saint Thomas Aquinas, René Descartes, and Immanuel Kant in Tom Regan and Peter Singer, eds., *Animal Rights and Human Obligations*, second edition (Englewood Cliffs: Prentice Hall, 1989).

posed difference in treatment in such a way as to render the double standard—treating all humans one way and all nonhuman animals another—defensible. But when the difference in treatment concerns the infliction of physical pain, it would appear that Bentham had it right: "the question is not, Can they reason? Nor, Can they talk? But, Can they suffer?"[10]

It would be wrong to conclude from this that we should always look to mere sentience, as opposed to linguistic capacity, or rationality, or some other advanced ability, in deciding the moral limits on how we may treat others. The point, rather, is that there is no single feature, or single cluster of features, that is always exhaustively relevant in determining how a given being should be treated in a given situation. The characteristics that are relevant to one situation are not always those that are relevant to another, so one cannot point to any single set of characteristics that some beings, but not others, might share, and declare them the unique and sufficient determiners of moral status. In deciding which applicant to hire for the position of lifeguard, swimming ability is relevant, but advanced knowledge of the law is not. In deciding which candidate to hire for associate attorney in a law firm, the identities of the relevant and irrelevant considerations are reversed. And if any of these applicants for jobs at the swimming pool or law firm show up at the emergency room in the hospital, they should be treated not in accordance with their swimming abilities or knowledge of the law but rather on the basis of the nature of their illnesses or injuries. The obvious conclusion to be drawn from these examples is, in James Rachels's words, that "before we can determine whether a difference between individuals is relevant to justifying a difference in treatment, we must know what sort of treatment is at issue," since "there is no one big difference between individuals that is relevant to justifying all differences in treatment."[11]

---

[10] Jeremy Bentham, from *The Principles of Morals and Legislation*, Chapter 17, Section 1, in Regan and Singer, *Animal Rights and Human Obligations*, p. 26.

[11] James Rachels, *Created from Animals* (New York: Oxford University Press, 1990), pp. 177–78. Notice that this argument against arbitrary double standards raises questions about the morality of killing animals for food, and not merely about the practice of doing so in an excessively cruel manner. After all, few would defend the painless killing of even the least mentally competent human beings for food, especially when plant-based foods, adequate to meet all of our nutritional needs, are abundantly available.

Intuition

In response to this argument, some defenders of meat eating, perhaps tacitly conceding that the search for features which both distinguish humans from animals and are relevant to justifying our use of animals as food is doomed to failure, have instead suggested that the rightness of assigning a privileged moral status to human beings is intuitively evident. According to this view, the thesis that we are morally superior to other animals, and that we consequently have the right to use them for food, possesses a kind of deep obviousness that renders argument unnecessary. At the very least it is claimed that this thesis exhibits a greater degree of intuitive obviousness than do any of the proposed arguments attempting to overturn it. For example, Jan Narveson objects that Tom Regan's defense of animal rights relies on "intuitions taken from the very set of received beliefs from which he is so considerably dissenting." Thus, since the results of Regan's analysis (for instance, that animals have rights and that vegetarianism is morally obligatory) are "rather unintuitive," Narveson suggests that we are free to draw upon "another selection" of intuitions, which would support our current practices.[12]

In response to Narveson, I will begin by conceding that moral vegetarianism does, perhaps, rely on intuited fundamental moral principles. We have already discussed one of these: that it is morally wrong to cause unnecessary pain. Another is a principle of equality or consistency: if it is wrong in one case to do X, then it will also be wrong to do so in another, unless the two cases differ in some morally relevant respect. It is this principle of equality or consistency that drives the demand that meat eaters must find some morally relevant difference between humans and other animals if they are to justify their practice. The reason is that all parties to the dispute agree that it would be wrong to slaughter human beings for the purpose of eating them. Consequently, this principle holds that it will also be wrong to treat animals this way unless animals differ from

---

[12] Jan Narveson, "On a Case for Animal Rights," *Monist* 70, No. 1 (January 1987), p. 48. See also C.A.J. Coady, "Defending Human Chauvinism," in Sylvan Barnet and Hugo Bedau, eds., *Current Issues and Enduring Questions*, second edition (Boston: Bedford, 1990), p. 265.

humans in some respect that is relevant to justifying the treatment in question. Defenders of moral vegetarianism cannot provide proof for these principles. That pain is generally a bad thing, that it hurts, is a basic datum of experience; and the principle of consistency appears to be a prerequisite to logic or coherent thought. But for those individuals, if there are any, who genuinely do not see that it is morally wrong to cause unnecessary pain, or that cases that are either identical or else differ only in irrelevant ways should be treated the same, I have no idea how one would go about convincing them. But Narveson claims the same for his principles—that humans are morally superior to animals, and that humans may use animals as food. He says that these principles, while incapable of being proved, are intuitively obvious. How, then, do we choose between these two competing sets of intuitive claims? Are they on equal footing? Must our choice between them be made simply arbitrarily, or perhaps on nonmoral grounds, such as those of self-interest?

I think not. I come down firmly on the side of the first set of intuitions, and I do not consider my choice the slightest bit arbitrary. By way of explanation, I offer three points. First, while it seems to me powerfully evident, from my own experience and from reflection on that experience, that happiness is intrinsically good and misery is intrinsically bad (or at least that happiness is intrinsically better than misery), I have no comparably strong intuition that human interests should be granted a privileged moral status in comparison to animals' interests. For when I reflect on my experientially grounded sense of the badness of my misery, it appears to me quite clearly that the badness flows from the nature of the misery, rather than from the fact that I am the one experiencing the misery. To be sure, the fact that I am the one experiencing the misery explains why I am the one who is intimately aware of this particular case of badness. But the misery appears to me to be bad as such—something that would be bad for whoever experienced it, including, for example, a pig. Of course, one might present some argument for the conclusion that it is not nearly so bad a thing for a pig to experience the sort of misery that it clearly is a bad thing for me to experience. But this would require argument. Since what is clearly given in my experience of misery is that misery as such is seriously bad, the burden of proof is on those who would claim that sometimes it is not. Given this burden of proof, intuition, in the absence of argument, will not suffice.

My second point in support of the first set of intuitions stems from the observation that one of the chief practical dangers attaching to any appeal to intuition concerns the ever-present possibility that one is confusing the intuitively evident with the merely familiar or the culturally given. Narveson notes this problem, observing, correctly, that "received moral views . . . don't come stamped with 'Genuine' and 'Culturally Biased' labels," and concludes, on that basis, that defenders of animal rights should leave him alone to "continue to eat meat in good conscience" until they can explain why they favor one set of intuitions over another.[13] But while Narveson is right to point out that cultural factors can distort our sense of what is and is not intuitively obvious, it doesn't seem to occur to him that, mindful of this danger, we might, through thoughtful inquiry, make some progress in distinguishing "genuine" intuitions from "culturally biased" counterfeits. Accordingly, I submit that my experientially grounded conclusion that happiness is intrinsically better than misery flourishes independently of cultural support and, indeed, would flourish in the face of cultural opposition. For happiness and misery do not present themselves with the kind of plasticity or flexibility necessary for their evaluation to be strongly susceptible to cultural manipulation. This does not seem to me to be the case with regard to the issue of the degree of importance to which considerations of animals' interests should be given in our moral deliberations. Consider that, while it would be quite shocking to learn of a culture in which misery is greatly prized for its own sake, it does not even surprise us to read of cultures which assign to animals a radically different moral status, whether higher or lower, than that which we assign to them.

Finally, I would point out that while our opposed fundamental judgments—that misery as such is bad and that it is seriously bad only when suffered by humans—are both widely held, it is possible in the case of the latter, but not the former, to explain the popularity of the judgment by appealing to something other than its evidentness. I refer to the simple point that the latter judgment, unlike the former, is self-serving, benefiting

[13] Narveson, "On a Case for Animal Rights," pp. 47–48.

the relatively powerful humans who make the judgment, at the expense of the relatively powerless animals, who have no say in the matter and who suffer the consequences.

It would seem, then, that neither argument nor intuition can establish that it is morally justified to slaughter and eat animals, given our agreement that it would be wrong to treat human beings in that way. For, if my arguments are sound, there is no set of features that both distinguishes human from other animals and does so in a way that relevantly justifies using one of these groups for food while scrupulously refraining from so using the other group. Nor can the appeal to intuition to justify our current practices succeed, since the thesis that humans are of vastly greater moral worth than other animals is manifestly less intuitively evident than are the theses that generate the demand for justification of meat eating (for instance, the principle that pain is generally bad, that the infliction of unnecessary pain is wrong, and that double standards require justification). What little intuitive force the former thesis does possess can, unlike the theses which oppose it, be explained away as the result of cultural bias, familiarity, and self-interest.

Tradition

Some may object, however, that my dismissive stance with regard to cultural bias betrays a lack of sympathy for the way in which many people consider "the merely familiar" and "the culturally given" to be valuable in themselves. Thus, even if I am correct in rejecting the claim that the rightness of meat eating is intuitively evident, perhaps it can be more straightforwardly defended on traditionalist grounds. To insist that we give up meat is to demand that we abandon cherished traditions, renounce the practices of our parents, and strike out in a new, perhaps "unnatural," direction, at odds with the way things have been since time immemorial. Surely that's asking too much.

In reply, I'll limit myself to two points. First, while the traditional nature of a given practice may well serve as a legitimate reason, for persons with inclinations or tastes in that direction, to choose that practice over newer, nontraditional, alternatives, surely that is not the case when the newer practice is otherwise demonstrably superior in comparison to its traditional competitor. To think otherwise is to reject all change, and with it, all progress. After all, it was once traditional and customary, when traveling from the east coast of North America to the west coast, to do so on the back of a horse. More to the point, many atrocities (for example, the institution of slavery and the subordination of women) have been justified as traditional and customary practices. In short, while there is nothing wrong with having a fondness for tradition, and for choosing to engage in traditional activities in part for the reason that they are traditional, the fact that a practice is traditional says nothing about its acceptability from a moral standpoint. And if a practice is morally indefensible, its status as such cannot be overridden simply on the grounds that it is traditional.

Secondly, an appeal to tradition is especially unhelpful to the defender of the Atkins Diet. In the first place, notice that the title, "Dr. Atkins' New Diet Revolution," hardly suggests that Dr. Atkins is recommending his diet on the grounds that it is an old cherished tradition. Rather, he presents it as a "revolutionary" diet, a breakthrough, based on the latest scientific knowledge. Granted, he also claims that his diet is very much in keeping with the way in which people ate in pre-agricultural times, but he does so in the context of marshalling evidence in support of the diet's health-bestowing properties. He is not urging people to eat his way out of respect for the ways in which their parents taught them to eat, or so as to continue the practices that are common in their culture. To the contrary, he urges them to reject what their parents taught them about diet and nutrition, to turn their back on their culture's dominant dietary practices, and to embrace his diet instead because scientific evidence (allegedly) shows it to be better from the standpoint of nutrition and overall health. But notice that if an Atkins defender chooses to embrace this "revolutionary" diet on grounds of its alleged health-giving superiority, he or she cannot at the same time consistently appeal to tradition to turn away arguments attempting to demonstrate its moral inferiority.

Similarly, while eating animal flesh is indeed traditional in most cultures, modern factory farming methods clearly are not. Thus, the vast majority of meat-eating Atkins dieters—those who buy their meat at grocery stores and at restaurants, as opposed to acquiring their meat exclusively through hunting or from small family farms—are supporting economically a relatively new, nontraditional, and decidedly cruel, practice. They can't consistently justify doing so by appealing to tradition.

One Last Shot for Dr. Atkins

Some Atkins advocates might challenge my arguments by asserting that they underestimate the potential benefits of the Atkins approach. They might concede that the Atkins Diet would indeed stand condemned as cruel if it were merely one good way among others to lose weight. But Dr. Atkins's more zealous advocates claim that it is much more than that. They assert that it is vital for their health, and perhaps even necessary to it. They believe that the Atkins Diet, carried out over a lifetime, offers them their best (or perhaps their only) chance to be healthy, strong, and alert. And these, clearly, are fundamental, rather than trivial, goods. If it is necessary that animals suffer so that these goods may be attained, that is regrettable, to be sure. Steps should be taken to minimize this suffering, if possible. But it is unreasonable to ask human beings to jeopardize their health in order to protect animals from suffering.

In response, it must be pointed out, first of all, that, at least for the great majority of people, there is no evidence that the adoption of a vegetarian diet would pose any risk to their health. In fact, the evidence points in the opposite direction. For example, during World War I, between October 1917 and October 1918, a British blockade of Denmark prevented the importation of meat. The Danes were forced during this period to live on a vegetarian diet. During this same period the death rate in Denmark dropped by 34 percent. There had been no remotely comparable drop in the death rate for any similar period of time over the course of the previous eighteen years. When the blockade was lifted and the people returned to their "normal" and "traditional" meat-based diet, their death rate also returned to its normal and traditional level.[14]

Similarly, William Castelli, M.D., director of the Framingham Heart Study (the longest-running epidemiological study in medical history, administered by the National Heart, Lung, and Blood

---

[14] John Lawrence Hill, *The Case for Vegetarianism* (Lanham: Rowman and Littlefield, 1996), pp. 82–83.

Institute), concludes: "Vegetarians have the best diet. They have the lowest rates of coronary disease of any group in the country. . . . They have a fraction of our heart attack rate and they have only 40 percent of our cancer rate. On the average, they outlive other people by about six years now."[15] Little wonder, then, that even the conservative American Dietetic Association, in its official position paper on vegetarian diets, notes:

> Scientific data suggest positive relationships between a vegetarian diet and reduced risk for several chronic degenerative diseases and conditions, including obesity, coronary artery disease, hypertension, diabetes mellitus, and some types of cancer. . . . It is the position of The American Dietetic Association (ADA) that appropriately planned vegetarian diets are healthful, nutritionally adequate, and provide health benefits in the prevention and treatment of certain diseases.[16]

It seems highly unlikely, then, that a switch from the Atkins Diet to a carefully planned and rigorously followed vegetarian diet would result in seriously negative health consequences. Thus, even on the generous assumption that the Atkins Diet is the very best, the very healthiest, diet for a human being to follow, its benefit, against which one would have to weigh the disvalue of animal suffering that it produces, would not simply be "good health," but rather, and more precisely, the margin by which one's health is better on the Atkins Diet than it would be on the best vegetarian alternative. Now, Americans consume, on average, fifty-one pounds of chicken every year, fifteen pounds of turkey, sixty-three pounds of beef, forty-five pounds of pork, one pound of veal, and one pound of lamb.[17] Atkins dieters, one would presume, consume even more meat than this. The question, then, is not whether the killing of animals on such a scale is justified if it is necessary for human health, but rather whether

---

[15] William Castelli, M.D., as quoted in "Veg for Health," *Veg for Life: A Farm Sanctuary Campaign*, at: http://www.vegforlife.org/health.htm (accessed 20th March, 2005).

[16] "Position of the American Dietetic Association: Vegetarian Diets," *The Vegetarian Resource Group*, at: http://www.vrg.org/nutrition/adapaper.htm (accessed 20th March, 2005).

[17] Scully, *Dominion*, p. 322, quoting U.S. Department of Agriculture statistics from 1998.

it is justified if it is necessary for the production of some measure of good health over and above that which can be achieved on a vegetarian diet. I would argue that it is not, especially when one considers that, under the gruesome conditions of factory farming, such killing is itself typically an occasion for the infliction of significant suffering, and almost always is the termination of a life that has been characterized by little but such suffering.

An Atkins dieter might respond that this argument rightly condemns only factory farming methods, and not meat-eating as such. Accordingly, what is needed is not vegetarianism, but rather factory farm reform. But in reply it should be noted that factory farm methods are driven by economics, not sadism, and thus are unlikely to change anytime soon. If they were to change, the result would be a dramatic increase in the cost of meat, making an Atkins-style diet beyond the economic means of all but the very rich. And while it would indeed be a step in the right direction for committed Atkins enthusiasts to refrain scrupulously from eating factory farm–produced meat, the fact remains that increased adoption of the Atkins Diet in the current climate translates to increased consumption of such meat, rendering Atkins advocacy morally problematic (even leaving aside ethical questions about the nonpainful killing of animals for unnecessary human purposes).

Finally, for those who are unmoved by ethical appeals on behalf of animals, or for those who truly believe that they would be sick or miserable (or quickly dead) if they were to adopt a vegetarian diet (or abandon the Atkins Diet), consider the effects of meat-eating on other people:

> Most estimates conclude that plant foods yield about ten times as much protein per acre as meat does. . . . [An] acre of oats produces six times the calories yielded by pork, the most efficient of the animal products. . . .The implications of all this for the world food situation are staggering. In 1974 Lester Brown of the Overseas Development Council estimated that if Americans were to reduce their meat consumption by only 10 percent for one year, it would free at least 12 million tons of grain for human consumption—or enough to feed 60 million people."[18]

---

[18] Singer, *Animal Liberation*, pp. 165–66. See also Hill, *The Case for Vegetarianism*, Chapter 5, "The Argument from World Hunger."

Indeed, even the staunchest defenders of meat eating usually concede that meat is an inefficient source of calories, and even of protein. Accordingly, they do not deny that a widespread switch to vegetarianism would lead to an increase in the world's food supply. But they do deny that this fact implies that such a switch would ameliorate the world hunger problem. The reason is that the world's present food supply, if distributed reasonably equitably, would be sufficient to feed everyone.

But this argument overlooks the fact that a significant worldwide conversion to vegetarianism would greatly improve the distribution of food to the world's poor, and not merely increase the supply of food. The main reason for this is simply that there is an economic competition for grain fields, and it is almost always won by the wealthy (who can afford meat), and not by the poor (who cannot). A large percentage of agriculture in the developing world is put to raising animals for export to the wealthy countries. Millions go hungry while land that could be used for the production of plant food, right where they live, is instead used for grazing. And cereal products that could be used to feed these starving millions is instead fed to cattle and other livestock, as this satisfies the appetite of the wealthy for meat and maximizes profits for those in the business of agriculture. If the market for meat in the wealthy countries were to disappear, farmers in the developing nations would return to the production of plant-based food, which they would have to sell at a much lower price, thus facilitating better distribution to the poor.[19]

And just as a meat-based diet exacerbates the world hunger problem, so does it contribute to the destruction of our environment. "A pound of meat requires fifty times as much water as an equivalent quantity of wheat. . . . Dutch farms produce 94 million tons of manure a year, but only 50 million can safely be absorbed by the land. . . . The excess . . . is dumped on the land where it pollutes water supplies and kills the remaining natural

[19] See Hill, *The Case for Vegetarianism*, Chapter 5, "The Argument from World Hunger," and John Robbins, *May All Be Fed* (New York: Morrow, 1992) for further elaboration of the ways in which large-scale vegetarianism would lead to more equitable distribution of food.

[20] Singer, *Animal Liberation*, pp. 167–68. See also Hill, *The Case for Vegetarianism*, Chapter 4, "The Argument from Global Ecology."

vegetation in the farming regions of the Netherlands."[20] Moreover, the main cause of deforestation, both historically and today, is the desire to graze animals. This exacerbates the greenhouse effect and contributes to global warming. "The prodigious appetite of the affluent nations for meat means that agribusiness can pay more than those who want to preserve or restore the forests. We are, quite literally, gambling with the future of our planet—for the sake of hamburgers."[21]

So, even on the generous (and to my mind highly dubious) assumption that the Atkins Diet is more conducive to human health than are even the best vegetarian alternatives, its cost, in comparison to those alternatives, includes (1) significantly greater animal suffering and killing, (2) a worsening of the horrific global hunger problem, and (3) an accelerated destruction of the natural environment, which in turn poses many health risks to human beings. It's hard to imagine what sorts of advantages the Atkins Diet could possibly deliver to those wealthy enough to follow it that could be sufficient to justify the hardships it visits on everyone else (animals, the undernourished people of the world, and, in connection with environmental issues, all of us). It's even harder to imagine that it actually delivers such benefits, even on the assumption (which I concede to be a reasonable one) that it does benefit some people. I think it is easier to imagine a future world in which vegetarianism is the norm, and in which history teachers are faced with the daunting challenge of explaining to school children why their ancestors actually thought it was okay to kill animals in order to eat their flesh.

---

[21] Singer, *Animal Liberation*, pp. 168–69.

13

Warning—This Diet Is Not for Everyone: The Atkins Diet's Ecological Side Effects

STAN COX and MARTY BENDER

The Atkins debate is chock full of meat and potatoes, bellies and thighs, arteries and kidneys. Biology provides the weaponry in battles over the Atkins Diet, but the landscape being fought over is largely philosophical.

In recent decades, biology has become permeated with the centuries-old philosophy of reductionism—that is, the belief that we can understand a whole system by understanding or manipulating its individual parts. The Atkins Diet is precisely the sort of scheme one would expect reductionist scientific thought to produce: a simple biological ruse that deprives the body of carbohydrates, forcing it to generate energy by breaking down the fat and protein in its own tissues, through a metabolic process called ketosis. And slim, satisfied customers are living proof that the diet can succeed—at least for some people, for varying lengths of time—given that success is measured in a single dimension, on the bathroom scales.

Of course, if reductionism's main assumption doesn't hold—if the whole really is not the same as the sum of its parts—we're in for some surprises when we step back and look at the entire system. Here, we will attempt to escape that reductionist trap (an ambition never to be fully realized) via the ecological route. We will show that the Atkins Diet—a product of human ingenuity designed to address a uniquely human health problem—is hazardous to the health of a planet whose ecosphere is already being exploited well beyond its capacity.[1]

[1] M. Wackernagel, N.B. Schulz, D. Deumling, A.C. Linares, M. Jenkins, V.

Most of today's approaches to problem solving are rooted in philosophies that evolved in an "empty world,"[2] that is, a world in which human activities could draw on a seemingly limitless supply of biological and mineral resources and could send wastes out into an apparent void where they would never again be encountered. Explicitly challenging that world view are disciplines such as environmental ethics and ecological economics, which work on the premise that in recent decades we have come to live in a "full world,"[3] or at least in a world that is rapidly filling up. That has forced us, for the first time ever, to face the possibility that what we do today may undermine the planetary life-support system for our descendants and those of other species. And it raises philosophical questions: How far into the future does our obligation to future generations extend? Would we accept a descent into universal misery and maybe even human extinction, say, ten thousand years from now, but not in the year 2100? What about the year 3000? Even if we agree on an answer to those questions, we cannot choose with any confidence—given our current state of knowledge—an optimum political, economic, and social path that will keep our species going for the desired number of centuries or millennia.

Despite such uncertainties, ecologically-minded thinkers have latched onto "sustainability" as the yardstick by which to evaluate human activities. In probably no other discipline is there such widespread accord regarding the principal criterion for comparing courses of action.

Agreement on the importance of sustainability has been the easy part. Attempts to define it have reached nothing remotely resembling a consensus. First, because any attempt to satisfy human needs inevitably and irreversibly consumes resources, degrades the ecosphere, and produces wastes,[4] "sustainability" is not open ended. Nothing can be sustained forever, so an arbitrary time frame must be chosen. Secondly, sustainability is a

---

Kapos, C. Monfreda, J. Loh, N. Myers, R. Norgaard, and J. Randers, "Tracking the Ecological Overshoot of the Human Economy," *Proceedings of the National Academy of Sciences* 99 (2002), pp. 9266–271.

[2] Herman E. Daly and Joshua Farley, *Ecological Economics: Principles and Applications* (Washington, D.C.: Island Press, 2004), pp. 111–122.

[3] *Ibid.*

[4] Nicholas Georgescu-Roegen, *The Entropy Law and the Economic Process* (Cambridge, Massachusetts: Harvard University Press, 1971).

property of entire societies, or even of all human activity planet wide, which makes it impossible to evaluate or predict. Therefore, we are compelled to play the reductionist's role and ask whether individual phenomena—for example, the Atkins Diet—contribute to sustainability or undermine it.

In the absence of a widely accepted definition of sustainability (either global or particular), we will in this chapter follow Kant's admonition to "act only according to that maxim by which you can at the same time will that it should become a universal law."[5] That is, we will ask, "If all potential dieters on earth wanted to adopt the Atkins plan, would this be possible? In other words, is it conceivable that the earth could sustain a world full of Atkins dieters?"

To label as unsustainable any individual action that could not be sustained universally is a highly conservative approach; clearly, we can envision "sustainable" societies in which one may pursue activities that would not be possible for everyone, while perhaps compensating with restraint in other areas. On the other hand, the advantages of the universalizing criterion are that: (1) it is more likely to result in global sustainability—given our unpredictable future—than are less conservative approaches that depend on just the right balance being struck, and (2) it incorporates global fairness, in that no one may do what could not be done by everyone. Furthermore, it is difficult to determine the degree to which any specific activity is sustainable, whereas it is not hard to identify one that is unsustainable. That is because an apparently sustainable action may cease to be so if we follow its ripple effects outward far enough in space and time, whereas such widening ripples will not turn an unsustainable action into a sustainable one.

In weighing the relative importance of personal and collective action, environmentalists are constantly running up against dilemmas, many of them quite immediate and concrete (for example, "Would my testimony in Congress to protect an endangered species justify the vast quantity of fuel I'd have to consume to get to Washington in time?"). There is no more personal decision than the choice of the food and drink that one swal-

---

[5] Immanuel Kant, *Groundwork for the Metaphysics of Morals* (New Haven: Yale University Press, 2002), p. 14.

lows. Therefore, in weighing the Atkins Diet, we will be implicitly lending support to the view that universal problems (and their solutions) can be created by an accumulation of decisions made independently by innumerable people. But we will then widen our field of vision to examine a food-production system under which millions of us have come to regard one of life's basic necessities—food—as an enemy of good health. As soon as we do that, we will see that individual decision-making explains very little.

Taking Atkins Global

Throughout history and for most of the world's people today, animal-derived foods have been regarded as a luxury, because their production requires more resource consumption than does the growing of food crops. The Worldwatch Institute[6] reports that it takes sixty-eight times as much water to produce a pound of beef as it does to produce a pound of bread flour, and that animal protein is eight times costlier than plant protein in terms of fossil-fuel energy. The industrialized West has managed to put meat and dairy consumption within reach of even the most impoverished citizen, but only by drawing on vast reserves of soil, water, and energy.

To the extent that the Atkins Diet can help people shed unwanted weight, it may be of benefit to individuals and, it can be argued, to society as a whole. But here we have decided to ask a different question: "Could it be practiced universally?" For example, a physician might well ponder the long-term burden to be borne by health-care systems if every person who wanted to lose weight were to adopt the Atkins Diet, ingesting large quantities of protein and fat that might damage the heart, kidneys, and other organs. An ethicist might ask whether hundreds of millions of Western people, who already consume more than their share of the world's resources, should adopt a diet that leads them to indulge even more lustily in foods that the majority of their fellow humans can afford to eat only sparingly if at all. Likewise, it is appropriate that agricultural scientists attempt to predict the likely environmental consequences of universalizing the Atkins weight-loss program.

---

6 "Eating Meat," *World Watch* 17, No. 4 (2004), pp. 12–19.

One of philosophy's more versatile tools is the *thought experiment*: reasoning about "an imaginary scenario with the aim of confirming or disconfirming some hypothesis or theory."[7] We will now apply this method as we weigh the hypothesis that the Atkins Diet could be practiced universally *and* sustainably. Thought experiments can be classified in a myriad of ways; ours might be called a scientific, or "factive,"[8] experiment that has a philosophical aim. In examining the possible ecological consequences of a universal Atkins Diet, we cannot begin to anticipate all of the interacting causes and effects; however, we can attempt to trace the gross outlines of a planet on which humanity has fully embraced the low-carb idea.

The first step is to estimate the number of potential dieters. We'll start with the Worldwatch Institute's estimate that one billion of Earth's inhabitants are overweight[9]—a rough and debatable figure, we admit—and assume that on average they eat 56 grams of animal protein a day before starting on the Atkins Diet. (That is the average animal protein consumption in Western countries, and most people who decide they need to lose weight have been eating at a Western nutritional level.) If they all were to adopt the Atkins Diet, their requirement for animal protein would rise to about 100 grams.[10] To allow a billion dieters to claim an even bigger share of the world's current pro-

[7] Tamara Szabó Gendler, "Thought Experiments," *Encyclopedia of Cognitive Science* (New York: Routledge, 2002), p. 388.

[8] *Ibid.*, p. 389.

[9] Gary Gardner and Brian Halweil, "Underfed and Overfed: The Global Epidemic of Malnutrition." Worldwatch Paper #150 (Washington, D.C.: Worldwatch Institute, 2000).

[10] Western diets contain a daily average of about 100 grams of protein, 56 grams of which is animal-derived. We're assuming that on the Atkins Diet, the remaining 44 grams will also come from animal sources. This is reasonable for the initial phases of the diet (in which almost no calories may come from carbohydrates) as well as for the long-term maintenance phase. In the maintenance phase, carbohydrate intake is generally limited to a range of 50 to 100 grams—about what you'd get in a serving of pasta. Very few vegetable-derived foods are low enough in carbohydrates to fulfill that requirement. That implies a lifelong need to get the bulk of one's daily calories from animal-derived foods. Dr. Atkins himself did not believe his diet was for vegetarians: "In general, I've found that a person who will not eat any animal foods will not do Atkins permanently. They find it too boring." R.C. Akins, *Dr. Atkins' New Diet Revolution* (New York: Avon, 2002), p. 149.

duction would be neither fair nor feasible, when that group of people already consumes more than twice as much animal protein per capita as the rest of humanity. Therefore, if we were to supply these new Atkins disciples with an extra 44 grams of animal protein each day, we'd need to boost overall production.

With some rough calculations, we can predict that that increase would be steep. The current human population of about 6.5 billion people consumes approximately 182 billion grams of animal protein per day. Therefore, supplying an additional 44 billion grams would require that the world's meat, dairy, poultry, and seafood industries increase their output by 25 percent.

The Atkins dieters would no longer get much of their protein from plant sources (grains being too heavily "polluted" with carbohydrates), so somewhat less land would be required for producing food crops. Still, the net result of their big switch to animal protein would require almost 250 million more acres[11] for corn, soybeans, and other feed grains. That's because feeding grain to animals and then eating the resultant meat, milk, eggs, or farm-raised fish is much less efficient than eating plant products directly.

Finding a quarter-billion acres for adequate feed-grain harvests would mean at least a 7 percent increase in cropland worldwide, at a time when farmers are already using just about all of the better land. Much of the newly plowed acreage would likely be marginal, prone to greater erosion, and in need of extra-generous applications of fertilizers and pesticides.

Furthermore, a livestock population explosion would worsen the air- and water-pollution crisis already being created by feedlots, poultry and hog confinement operations, and slaughterhouses. Trying to spare the land and squeeze more protein from the already overfished oceans would likely be even more damaging.

And that's not all. Cattle and other ruminant animals obtain a large share of their food from pasture and rangeland. Were their

---

[11] A 25-percent increase in animal populations would require almost 500 million additional acres for feed grain production. Meanwhile, with a billion dieters shunning plant-based foods, 250 million acres less would be needed for production of food crops. Therefore, 500 – 250 = a 250 million-acre net increase in cropland.

numbers to increase by 25 percent, current grasslands probably could not bear the entire burden. Most of those lands are already fully stocked, and putting more animals on them would result in an even higher rate of overgrazing and degradation. If new pastures were to be created for, say, half of the additional animals, a billion more acres would have to be found. Most of this additional grassland would probably be created by deforestation, which could mean that 10 percent of the Earth's remaining forests would have to go.

Overconsumption in America and other affluent nations doesn't exactly qualify as breaking news, but the Atkins Diet puts a new twist in the old story. Its advocates have convinced millions of people that the most effective way to reduce the size of their own bodies is to gobble up global resources at an even faster rate.

The Bigger Picture

Now, we realize that in practice every potential dieter on the planet is not going to adopt the Atkins program. Many people are happy with their weight the way it is, and a significant proportion of those who do want to shed pounds lack the financial means to make expensive animal-based products their primary food source. Furthermore, debates over the diet's soundness remain unresolved. Surveys show that the popularity of low-carb dieting appears to have peaked in mid-2004 and may even be on the decline.[12] Nevertheless, the kinds of ecological damage we have described are likely to occur in direct proportion to the number of people who do follow the Atkins plan, and that information should be placed on the scales when one is weighing the costs and benefits of various diets.

To this point, we have left unexamined a major assumption of our thought experiment. In concluding that ecological damage would be likely to occur with further growth of the Atkins empire, we assumed that our expanded bovine populations would eat a grain-based diet for much of their lives, as do the vast majority of American cattle today. Half of all grain in the

---

[12] Johanna Crosby, "Has the Low-Carb Craze Crashed?" *Cape Cod Times* (20th January, 2005): http://www.capecodonline.com/cctimes/health/lowcarb20.htm.

U.S. is fed to animals. Sixty percent of that portion goes to beef and dairy cattle, with most of the remaining feed grains being used to produce pork and poultry.

But with alternative production systems, moderate beef consumption could actually help improve the environment. Cattle, unlike chickens and hogs, can subsist almost entirely on range, pasture, and hay. Extensive research shows that rangelands and pastures, which are dominated by perennial plants with large, long-lived root systems, do not generate the high levels of soil erosion and water contamination seen in annual grain crops. Therefore, we could dramatically improve the state of this continent's lands and rivers by taking the 60 percent of feed-grain acreage that currently goes to cattle and converting it to pasture. Were that done, our calculations show that production of beef and dairy products might be maintained at current levels; however, output probably could not be raised to a level at which it could supply a universally adopted Atkins Diet, unless we were to create expansive new grasslands through deforestation.

Back here in the real world, Atkins-inspired increases in beef demand are being met largely by stuffing corn and soybean meal into feedlot-raised cattle. Unfortunately, the Corn Belt will not become a more ecologically friendly Range and Pasture Belt in the foreseeable future. In an American economy groaning under huge grain surpluses, cattle are prized, ironically, for their *in*efficiency—that is, for their ability to convert ten pounds of unneeded corn into only one pound of meat. That shrinkage of the food supply serves an important economic function, given our dysfunctional economy. It will take sweeping changes, going far beyond shifts in personal diet, to make America's meat industry more ecologically sound.

When all factors are considered, diet regimens that emphasize plant products are more likely to be ecologically universalizable than are regimens based on animal protein. And it is possible, with considerable ingenuity and effort, to achieve the Atkins-recommended intake of protein, fat, carbohydrates, and fiber on a vegetarian diet. Few, if any, plant-derived foods in their native state can satisfy those requirements, so vegetarian low-carb diets are necessarily heavy in isolated, processed vegetable proteins. But the Atkins Diet has owed its popularity to the very *absence* of just such foods; a low-carb dieter relaxing on her patio, grilling a T-bone, is unlikely to yearn for texturized vegetable protein. Only if you're a deeply committed vegetarian could you feel that you're eating "the foods you love" on a plant-based Atkins Diet. Eco-conscious low-carb dieters who expend time, energy, and, above all, money in seeking out grass-fed beef or soy sausage are to be applauded. But would even those routes to weight loss be universally fair and sustainable? To follow any highly selective diet is to exercise a privilege typically reserved for the few. Graham Greene put it best in his novel *The Comedians*, when Mr. Brown, the narrator, consoles the altruistic Mr. Smith regarding Smith's failed proposal for a "vegetarian center" in Haiti: "I don't think they are quite ripe here for vegetarianism. Perhaps you must have enough cash to be carnivorous first."

Atkins: Yet Another Metabolic Rift

Silvia Federici has shown[13] that seventeenth-century philosophers' deep interest in the human body as a mechanical contraption—particularly Descartes's view of the mind as separate from and in command of the mechanical body—opened the door to its exploitation through wage labor. Federici goes so far as to suggest that "the human body, and not the steam engine, and not even the clock, was the first machine developed by capital." Parallel to its usefulness as a producer of goods, the body-as-machine is, of course, an excellent consumer as well. Of that, there is no better example than the Atkins Diet. Walk the aisles of any supermarket, and it is clear that by simply tripping a metabolic switch in dieters, Atkins has not only increased resource consumption but also provided countless marketing opportunities.[14]

For comparison, let's pursue a second thought experiment. This time, all the people on the planet who want to lose weight follow a more commonly suggested route to better health. They follow these recommendations:

---

[13] Silvia Federici, "The Great Caliban: The Struggle Against the Rebel Body," *Capitalism Nature Socialism* 15, No. 2 (2004), pp. 7–16; "The Great Caliban: The Struggle Against the Rebel Body—Part 2," *Capitalism Nature Socialism* 15, No. 3 (2004), pp. 13–28. The quotation is from p. 18.

[14] For more on the issue of diets as a marketing opportunity, see Chapter 10 in this volume.

- Eat less.
- Eat out rarely.
- Cook using food in a less-processed form: for example whole-grain flour, eggs, poly- and monounsaturated oils, dry beans, home-grown vegetables, rolled oats, and so on.
- Limit consumption of animal products.
- Drink mainly water.
- Avoid between-meal snacks.
- Walk, run, or bike instead of driving whenever possible.

Heeding this prosaic advice may or may not result in weight loss, and it may or may not be ecologically sustainable. That depends on the many assumptions and variables that are submerged within it. But we can be confident that it would cause less environmental damage than current Western eating habits. Furthermore, it would tend not to generate friction between the rights of humans and those of other species; it would call attention to the ultimate dependence of humans on natural systems; it would be unlikely to run up against conflicts between personal responsibility and sociopolitical action; it would be more affordable for rich and poor alike; *and* it would probably trigger an economic collapse.

Were hundreds of millions of people to settle into such a routine, they would dam up the vast rivers of capital that currently go into agribusiness and the food industry. The global economy, as it exists today, owes it existence to uninterrupted growth in consumption. In that economy, a phenomenon like the Atkins Diet that opens up whole new vistas for capital accumulation is much to be preferred over, say, empty parking lots at McDonald's and Safeway.

As a way to protect and improve the condition of the human body, the Atkins Diet takes its place in a long parade of profitable but ecologically harmful products that displaced more benign activities. In recent decades, we've substituted workouts in upscale fitness clubs for a few hours of hauling hay bales; we've consumed pricey bottled water instead of formerly safe-to-drink tap water; we've fostered allergies and then alleviated them with drugs and air conditioning; and we've allowed the Atkins Diet to triumph over a balanced diet of whole foods that requires simple restraint. Design a product that combines luxury consumption with notions of health and vitality, and you can bet (sorry, Dr. Atkins) that it will sell like hotcakes.

Plans like Atkins that emphasize the ingestion not of food but of the individual compounds into which food can be broken—such as sugars, starches, proteins, fats, fiber, vitamins, antioxidants—are part of a larger trend that includes the booming nutritional-supplement market. This atomization of food is the latest in a series of "metabolic rifts" (to use the philosopher Karl Marx's term[15]) that have torn through agriculture in recent centuries.

The first rift came with the Industrial Revolution, as essential soil components like nitrogen, phosphorus, and organic matter began to be exported from the land in the form of food for city-dwellers, whose nutrient-rich waste products were then lost into the rivers and oceans.

In the early twentieth century, the discovery of a method for using fossil fuel to make nitrogen fertilizer provided a short-term fix for the soil-fertility crisis. But in the last two decades of the century, a second rift resulted from the rapid growth of feedlots and indoor animal-confinement operations. Animal husbandry and crop production, formerly woof and warp of the same agricultural fabric, were ripped from each other, creating further crises of pollution, soil degradation, and poor human nutrition.

Now the very concept of food is starting to fade away, as what we eat is regarded more and more as a simple agglomeration of nutrients in various proportions. Today it's low-carb oddities like bunless submarine sandwiches, crustless pizzas and pies, "mashed potatoes" made of isolated soy protein, breadless Thanksgiving stuffing, and, of course, pork rinds. Tomorrow, perhaps, we'll be popping the Jetsons' meal-in-a-pill.

With each successive rift in the networks that link soil, water, microbial communities, insects, wild plants, crops, livestock populations, and human beings, we have attempted to impose the factory model on living systems, with predictably ruinous consequences for the ecosphere. In his essay "The Pleasures of Eating,"[16] Wendell Berry writes that in freeing ourselves from the

---

[15] John Bellamy Foster, *Marx's Ecology: Materialism and Nature* (New York: Monthly Review Press, 2000), pp. 155–163.

[16] Wendell Berry, "The Pleasures of Eating," in *What are People For?* (New York: North Point Press, 1990).

hard work and restraint that characterize the agrarian world, we walked right into a trap. He then offers this advice:

> How does one escape this trap? Only voluntarily, the same way that one went in: by restoring one's consciousness of what is involved in eating; by reclaiming responsibility for one's own part in the food economy. One might begin with the illuminating principle of Sir Albert Howard's *The Soil and Health*, that we should understand "the whole problem of health in soil, plant, animal, and man as one great subject." Eaters, that is, must understand that eating takes place inescapably in the world, that it is inescapably an agricultural act, and how we eat determines, to a considerable extent, how the world is used. This is a simple way of describing a relationship that is inexpressibly complex. To eat responsibly is to understand and enact, so far as we can, this complex relationship.

In the world Berry envisions, low-carb diets would be about as compelling as ketchup on a homegrown tomato. And therein lies the key. We can't change the world for the better simply by debunking the Atkins Diet; on the contrary, the world will have to change dramatically before we see the end of food fads.

Part 5

Unlimited Noncaloric Beverages

(Cultural Intersections)

14
Men on Atkins: Dieting, Meat, and Masculinity

AMY BENTLEY

"You get to eat a ton of red meat." That's how most people respond when asked to describe the Atkins Diet. There's no question that Atkins is unusual, even compared to other popular low-carb diets, in that it prescribes, even encourages, the consumption of meat and other high-protein, high-fat animal-derived foods such as hard cheese, bacon, sour cream, pork rinds, and beef jerky. In fact, under Atkins what can be considered "diet food" has left many Americans scratching their heads: low-carb dieters consume large quantities of Atkins-sanctioned bacon and pork rinds now that pretzels, grapes, even the ubiquitous carrot stick—healthy snacks in the low-fat diet regimen—are considered off limits because they contain too many carbohydrates.

Meat, naked and unadorned, seems to be at the forefront of every low-carb meal, and it seems as if the entire food industry has shifted in part to cater to the "Atkins lifestyle." Fast-food joints, high-end restaurants, and everything in between have gone from removing the bread or pasta at an individual customer's request to creating menus featuring Atkins-like meal options. The "casual American dining" chain T.G.I. Friday's has partnered with Atkins to offer such Atkins-approved menu options as "Tuscan Spinach Dip and Buffalo Wings" and "Sizzling N.Y. Strip with Bleu Cheese."

Because of its emphasis on red meat the Atkins Diet takes on a strongly male persona, which has allowed men to come out of the dieting closet. Many men feel much more comfortable admitting to being on Atkins and other low-carb diets, unlike the more traditional low-fat diets that feature such "female" foods as fruits and vegetables, fish, grains, and low-fat dairy products. In fact, the whole widespread popularity of Atkins has had interesting implications for food in our culture, including the "masculinization" of dieting—or, at least, a tempering of its strongly traditional female connection.

Understanding Masculinity

"Masculinity" is one of those concepts that everyone understands but can't readily define. If you asked your teen-aged brother to describe what being masculine means, he might respond with something like, "It's not feminine." Or, "It's being a guy." Or, "It's liking trucks and guns and football, and not liking ballet and tear-jerker movies on the Lifetime channel." And in part he is right, since these crass generalizations begin to set up what is called the "hypermasculine" ideal construction of maleness: stereotyped ideas about being male and female that have little to do with biology but a lot to do with agreed-upon rules of what is "normal" in society.[1] Philosopher Patrick D. Hopkins has noted that when in high school, a football player would insult another by calling him a "girl." "Girl," explains Hopkins, "signifie[d] a failure of masculinity, a failure of living up to a gendered standard of behavior, and a gendered standard of identity."[2]

To explain a bit further, throughout most of history most societies, including our own Western culture, have been built on patriarchy. Men (at least those of the privileged class) have held more political power, have had more access to wealth, have been given more legal rights, and have had more opportunities for education. Men have been valued more highly than women; what is "male" has been regarded as "better" than what is "female."

---

[1] For a more detailed discussion, see John Stoltenberg, *Refusing to be a Man* (Portland: Breitenbush, 1989).

[2] Patrick D. Hopkins, "Gender Treachery: Homophobia, Masculinity, and Threatened Identities," in Larry May, Robert Strikwerda, and Patrick D. Hopkins, eds., *Rethinking Masculinity: Philosophical Explorations in Light of Feminism* (Lanham: Rowman and Littlefield, 1996), p. 96.

In fact, the idea of "masculine" has always been defined in opposition to and in dominance over what is regarded as female. One scholar of masculinity notes that the first rule of traditional American manhood has been "no sissy stuff: men can never do anything that even remotely suggests femininity. Manhood is a relentless repudiation of the feminine."[3] This is why homosexuality throws these stereotypical assumptions about masculinity into question, because it blurs, even destabilizes, the strict, prescriptive notions of masculine and feminine. Further, ideal notions of masculinity are under pressure for economic reasons. Given that a sense of masculinity has been linked to economic production, to being the family breadwinner, in the current economic climate of uncertainty it is impossible (and for many undesirable) for most men to "win the bread" solely by themselves.[4]

While these strict definitions and notions of female and male have largely diminished today, we can still see lingering remnants. Women wear pants in public; one rarely sees a man wearing a skirt. It seems more normal for a woman to like football, for instance, than it does for a man to like ballet or hopscotch. Similarly, a woman is usually regarded positively when pursuing the male-dominated field of engineering, while a man who willingly becomes a stay-at-home parent often faces questions over his masculinity. Because of the long-standing hierarchy of men over women, when women take on traditionally male-dominated professions they are elevating their status; conversely, when men assume traditionally female roles they are demeaning themselves by acting "womanish." Notions of gender-appropriate activities also include dieting, which has long been regarded as a female activity.

(Un)Manliness and Dieting

Body size and dieting nicely illustrate the concepts of masculinity and femininity. Since large size symbolizes power, throughout much of history the ideal body for men has depended in part on

---

[3] Michael Kimmel, "Clarence, William, Iron Mike, Magic—and Us," *Changing Men* (Winter–Spring 1993), pp. 9–10.

[4] Larry May and Robert A. Strikwerda, "Fatherhood and Nuturance," in *Rethinking Masculinity*, pp. 193–210.

being larger than women's, on having a greater physical presence. Though a muscular body is preferable to a rotund physique, men have traditionally been able to get away with a measure of portliness. By contrast, women are supposed to be smaller. Given the emphasis modern Western culture places on female slimness, along with the fact that the fundamental purpose of dieting is to deprive yourself in order to make yourself smaller, it is not surprising that since the early twentieth century in the United States dieting has always been thought of as a female activity.

Because of this, for a man to embrace dieting wholeheartedly potentially contained some element of threat to his masculinity; to declare publicly that he was dieting left a man open to possible ridicule about his virility. So while men in some number have always intentionally tried to lose weight, they traditionally have avoided publicly admitting to dieting in the same way as women. Of course this does not apply to all men equally. Gay men and so-called metrosexuals—heterosexual men who are comfortable engaging in traditionally female behaviors—may not have experienced this typecasting to the same extent as most heterosexual men, particularly those from the working class and from certain ethnicities. Similarly, for body builders, wrestlers, and other serious athletes who have always rigorously controlled food intake as part of their training, publicly discussing their dieting habits has been less threatening to their masculinity largely because their activities have marked them as especially masculine.

In the twenty-first century, both men and women still regard slimness as more important for women. Yet in today's world, where equality means in part that the popular media scrutinize men's and women's bodies alike, men are being subjected to, and are responding to, social pressures to maintain fit, lean (though muscular) bodies. Like women, they have turned to dieting as a way to achieve and maintain this body image, as well as to maintain health.

Enter Atkins

Atkins has helped to masculinize dieting, allowing men a greater level of comfort in the world of dieting.[5] Men on Atkins regu-

---

[5] Judith Weinraub, "Suddenly It's a Guy Thing; In the Beginning, Before Low-Carb

larly comment that what they value about the diet is how "easy it is to eat out." They do not have to feel self-conscious ordering a large piece of animal flesh as they might when ordering "just a salad." Not only do men feel more comfortable admitting they are on a diet, Atkins allows men to discuss dieting with enthusiasm. In fact, the discussion of a group of low-carb male dieters resembles "typical" female chitchat about food, dieting, and health: what to eat, what to avoid, what to do about portion sizes, what to do when clothing doesn't fit anymore, and so on. For many men dieting clearly has become a pleasurable topic of conversation.

I know of one all-male group of business-school professors at a prestigious university that has found a new camaraderie over low-carb dieting. While dining out together a year or so ago, they realized they all were following some form of low-carb/high-protein diet, with apparently great success. "We had all lost about thirty pounds," one related later. When the animated conversation turned to ordering, they decided collectively which high protein appetizers they would order to share among the group. Spurred on by their collective low-carb experience, the group, which one refers to as his "diet-talk friends," continues to discuss food, health, and dieting, trading stories and food tips, even keeping weight and exercise charts on their computers. Nearly all agreed that Atkins and other low-carb diets seemed particularly inviting to men. One has even prepared a somewhat tongue-in-cheek lecture for his MBA students comparing Japanese theories of work productivity to low-carb dieting; he feels comfortable enough to include a Power Point slide of his weight chart as part of the lecture.

Indeed, Atkins capitalizes on its male-friendly persona and does what it can to make its diet, its promotional materials and website, and its products accessible to men. For example, the Atkins website lists dozens of "success stories": photos and narratives of real people who have lost weight on Atkins. Of the forty-three recent Web profiles, nearly half are men, a high ratio when compared to the "success stories" at the Weight Watchers and Jenny Craig websites. Of the over two hundred stories

---

Eating, It Wasn't Manly to Watch your Weight," *Washington Post* (29th September, 2004), p. F1.

posted on the Jenny Craig website, only sixteen are men's. (Also contributing to the masculine persona of Atkins is its close identification with its founder, Dr. Robert C. Atkins. In fact, most of the high-protein gurus tend to be men, thus increasing the "male-friendliness" of low-carb dieting. Both Atkins and Arthur Agatston, M.D., of the South Beach Diet began their careers as cardiologists, one of the most masculine of medical specialties.)

Men profiled in the Atkins success stories often note that they heard about the diet from other men, or watched another man lose weight on Atkins, which made them willing to try it. For some, dieting commences as a competition against another male to lose weight. Terry Free, for example, writes: "In February of 2002, two friends told me they had started doing Atkins. I had never heard of it, but they were losing weight so I thought I'd give it a try. I asked another friend, who only needed to lose ten pounds, to try Atkins with me, if only for two weeks. 'Let's show these other two guys up,' I said. He agreed, so I went to the Atkins website and bought a copy of *Dr. Atkins' Diet Revolution*."[6] Similarly, Bob Keown explains, "[A]round the time of my thirty-sixth birthday, my wife had bumped into a guy she used to work with. He'd lost thirty pounds in three months doing Atkins. I bought *Doctor Atkins' New Diet Revolution* that afternoon."[7]

Food Has a Gender?

Atkins is popular with men in part because many of the foods the diet allows and even encourages its dieters to consume are stereotypically masculine. Meat, across cultures and throughout time, has been regarded as in the male domain. Some see this symbolic connection between meat and men in part the result of the legacy of hunter-gatherer days when men killed and brought home large game animals and then distributed them to the village. Women, by contrast, were traditionally responsible for trapping small game, fishing, gathering wild foods, and cultivating fruits and vegetables. While these food-gathering activi-

---

[6] Atkins Nutritionals, www.atkins.com, "A Successful Wager," http://atkins.com/Archive/2003/3/18-41314.html.

[7] Atkins Nutritionals, www.atkins.com, "Back in the Game," http://atkins.com/Archive/2001/12/21-882879.html.

ties no doubt accorded women their own measure of power, men controlled the high-status large, dangerous game meat, and accrued power because of it.

While meat has been squarely in the masculine category, traditional diet foods such as vegetables, fruit, fish, and low-fat salad dressings—and salads in general—have long been regarded as "female" foods. Nearly every culture symbolically associates gender with particular foods. In these cultural linkages, meat has most commonly been identified with men, and "nonmeats," especially grains, fruits, and sugars, with women. In Eastern thought, for example, the concepts of yin and yang associate meat with the masculine yang and fruits and vegetables with the feminine yin. As a child growing up in the United States I learned that little boys are made of such carnivorous delicacies as snails and puppy dog tails, while little girls are made of sugar and spice—everything "nice."[8]

These strong associations make it feel vaguely inappropriate to identify women with meat and even more strongly improper to associate men with, say, sugar or lettuce. If real men don't eat quiche, according to a popular 1970s phrase, they certainly should avoid "rabbit food." One male athlete friend of mine admitted, "Eating a steak sounds more masculine than eating carrots." Indeed, in contrast to the salads, steamed vegetables, and broiled fish of low-fat diets, the prototypical Atkins meal sounds like something right off a steakhouse menu, oozing with testosterone: bacon strips for an appetizer, then steak, creamed spinach, and a small salad with Caesar dressing—but hold the croutons, and ditto the foil-wrapped baked potato. "There occurred a weird power imbalance when my husband, dieting on Atkins, sat down across the table from me, a vegetarian, with his 'diet food' plate full of steak and hunks of cheese," a female friend related.

These strong symbolic associations are also due in part to the "you are what you eat" principle: the belief that people absorb characteristics of the foods they ingest, particularly animal flesh. In some cultures, for example, people believe eating the eyes of animals improves one's eyesight, or eating tortoise flesh produces

---

[8] For a thorough discussion of the symbolic meanings of meat see Nick Fiddes, *Meat: A Natural Symbol* (London: Routledge, 1991).

lethargy, or, in Western culture (as elsewhere), eating beef makes one "strong as an ox," a strongly masculine identification. This explains why many Americans regard a woman with a large piece of meat on her plate as less feminine than one eating a salad.

Yet strictly gendered notions of some foods may have softened, now that Atkins has deemed a big red steak diet food. To some extent Atkins makes meat safer for women to consume openly and with relish—something that has not always been the case. Over a decade ago psychologists found that both men and women regarded a woman eating a small salad and seltzer as more feminine, more socially appealing, and more attractive than the *same* woman eating heavier meals containing meat. While these perceptions no doubt still exist to some degree, restaurateurs are finding many more women ordering steaks and other large cuts of meat than just a few years ago, and the restaurateurs relate the change directly to Atkins. Women may enjoy partaking in this still fairly masculine act of consumption in a way they could not, for example, comfortably smoke an after-dinner cigar, which is still mostly deemed off-limits to women. While Atkins may be softening the stigma of women consuming meat in public, the relaxation of the even stronger taboo associating men with such "female" activity as dieting makes it the more prominent effect of the two.

Some men have mentioned that part of their attraction to Atkins had to do with the masculine foods Atkins emphasized. James Guilbeaux reveals that "I'm not a big vegetable guy, and that makes it hard to go on most diets."[9] One of Doug Berry's strategies for success is, "Any time you feel hungry or tempted, make yourself a great low carb meal like a juicy rib-eye steak with asparagus drenched with butter. How can you feel deprived when you can eat like this?"[10] Another man summed up his attraction to Atkins by noting, "It's a pretty cool diet. You can eat bacon and eggs and all kinds of great stuff, and get away with it."[11] By contrast, one woman who tried Atkins remarked of

---

[9] Atkins Nutritionals, www.atkins.com, "Surf and Turf," http://atkins.com/Archive/2002/8/14-510853.html.

[10] Atkins Nutritionals, www.atkins.com, "A Toast to Good Health," http://atkins.com/Archive/2002/11/19-211272.html.

[11] Quoted in Lisa Blank Fasig, "Retailers Happily Find that Atkins Dieters Worth Their Weight in Gold," *Cincinnati Business Courier* (29th September, 2003), www.cincinnati.bizjournals.com.

the experience, "I know it sounds stereotypical, but when I was on Atkins all I wanted was a big fruit salad."

Atkins, Masculinity, and Class

Atkins's central focus on meat has interesting implications concerning class as well as gender. A dieter following a strict Atkins regimen must give up (at least for the most part) a large number of foods, including many that are cheap, industrially processed, and mass-produced—think pretzels, cookies, chips, bread, and pasta. This restriction means that people of a more comfortable income level are more likely to go on Atkins. The added expense of the diet creates a barrier for those with lower incomes, including many ethnic minorities. Of the forty-three Atkins success stories on the Atkins website, for example, all except three—two African-Americans and one Latino couple—are Caucasian Americans. Yet at the same time Atkins grants a sort of special status to certain foods—pork rinds, bacon, beef jerky—that are best known as part of so-called white trash foods and foodways, a version of Southern Appalachian cooking that is stereotypically heavy on grease and pork products. Such Atkins staples as pork rinds, bacon, and beef jerky, along with a general enthusiasm for fat and a penchant for large portions, run contrary to bourgeois ideals of food and dining.

Indeed, a surprising consequence of Atkins is the mainstream emergence of pork rinds—the scraped, deep-fried skins of pigs (*chicharrones*) once favored only among southerners and Latinos. When during the 1988 presidential election the elder George Bush went on record as listing pork rinds as his favorite snack, commentators agreed that it was an attempt to gain favor with white, working-class southern men, the so-called Bubba vote (an older cousin of the Nascar Dad). For most Americans even aware of the existence of pork rinds, they elicit a certain amount of disgust; for those who practice religions prohibiting pork, pork rinds are not only unpalatable but inedible. Yet since 2000 pork rinds, along with beef jerky, have been the fastest growing products in the salty snack foods category, tapping into the market share traditionally held by potato and tortilla chips; in 2003 pork rind sales topped $840 million.[12] Atkins dieters

---

[12] Marla Dickerson, "Slim Down with . . . Pork Rinds?" *Denver Post* (8th August,

who miss the salty crunch of chips find solace in the sanctioned pork rinds. Middle-class Atkins enthusiasts buy cinnamon-flavored pork rinds by the case and use crushed pork rinds as a breading for fried chicken. One Yankee business executive told of always looking forward to his travels to the South where "every vending machine has a package of pork rinds." A university administrator told me of coming home to find her Atkins-dieting husband "sitting in a chair, drinking a scotch, and dipping pork rinds into sour cream for a snack. Before Atkins, he would have never done that." One journalist, commenting on the increase in pork-rind consumption, spotlights Sandy Clark, described as "female, white-collar, health-conscious, and Jewish—lousy demographics for peddling deep-fried pigskin." While consuming two bags of pork rinds a week Clark has lost seventeen pounds since starting Atkins.[13]

The end result is a complicated notion of class and food that allows these "white trash" foods to edge their way into upper-middle-class respectability. French theorist Pierre Bourdieu has shown that in the realm of food, "taste" in its broadest definition can be examined and identified in terms of class. A low-fat regimen, adequate and persistent exercise, and a lean body are representative of an upper-middle-class taste culture—"habitus," as Bourdieu terms it—providing those who can attain it a kind of cultural capital.[14] Thus, the recent popularity of Atkins among educated, economically successful Americans has begun to create a space for pork rinds and beef jerky in the landscape of mainstream American foodways.

Low Fat versus Low Carb

As Atkins and other low-carbohydrate diets challenge the primacy of traditional low-fat diets, what has emerged is a competing set of rules about dieting that challenge and parallel, without fully displacing, the traditional low-fat diet. In many respects the two sets of rules differ dramatically: One counts calories and fat grams; the other tracks carbohydrates, seeing

---

2000), p. A-2; www.porkrind.com.

[13] Dickerson, "Slim Down with . . . Pork Rinds?"

[14] Pierre Bourdieu, *Distinction* (Cambridge, Massachusetts: Harvard University Press, 1984), p. 197.

calories as at best secondary. One demonizes high-fat foods while the other outlaws high-carb foods. One encourages lots of fruits and vegetables prepared with little or no fat, the other deems most produce off limits and recommends that vegetables be prepared with fat or eaten in combination with animal foods. One throws out bacon and pork rinds, the other celebrates them. One preaches restraint and deprivation; the other gives the appearance of sanctioning abundance and excess. Overall, the rules of food consumption—what is celebrated, what is taboo, what is a diet staple, and the rules of eating—are strikingly different. One man formerly on Atkins remembered, "For a snack during the day I would go into a deli and buy a half-pound of pastrami and eat the whole package of meat, maybe with some mustard, right then and there."[15]

To stretch the comparison a bit further we might say that one approach personifies the feminine and the other embodies the masculine, although we all know men who gravitate to a low-fat diet and women who find low carb a more natural fit. Studies on gendered food and eating patterns point to the conclusion that while women are more likely to be characterized by what they don't eat (food restriction through dieting), men are more likely to be characterized by what they consume (heavier, more "masculine" foods).[16]

Clearly Atkins and other diets low in carbs and high in protein and fat have not replaced our traditional ways of eating, just as low-fat diets have not permanently altered Americans' eating habits. While Atkins has declined in popularity, it still maintains a substantial number of adherents, and it will be interesting to see the future effects of Atkins on culture, the environment, health, politics, and economics. Whatever these results, the popularity of Atkins is due in part to its masculine-friendly nature—built on large chunks of animal flesh, particularly red meat—the same high-status food that has traditionally stood for abundance, wealth, and power.

---

[15] Personal interviews.

[16] For more on gender, food, and the body, see Susan Bordo, *Unbearable Weight: Feminism, Western Culture, and the Body* (Berkeley: University of California Press, 1993).

15
Low-Carb Dieting and the Mirror: A Lacanian Approach to the Atkins Diet

FABIO PARASECOLI

Who's the Fairest of Them All?

How often do we look in a mirror? Every day, when we get up, we often catch ourselves staring at the sleepy-eyed face that we recognize as our own, with a mix of curiosity, boredom, and matter-of-factness that confirms to us the sometimes dubious fact that we do exist. We look awry at ourselves in the hallway mirror while rushing to work. We peek at ourselves as we walk past a shop window. We may even sneak a glance at ourselves while sipping a drink in our favorite bar, wondering how we got to have such a dismayed demeanor.

Our reflection is a constant, though not always welcome, presence throughout our lives. We all remember the endless time spent in front of mirrors while growing up, during those awkward teen years, trying to figure out the right look to be cool, and at total loss about why our parents did not make us cool enough.

Mirrors continue to haunt us as adults. After all, which of us is totally comfortable, at all times, with our reflection? Too frequently, it does not exactly match what the world around us promotes as acceptable or preferable. It is not only a question of clothes, hairstyles, or accessories. Our body itself frequently bothers us, to the point we end up perceiving it as some external burden imposed on our real self, that inner self that does not succeed in shining through the obtrusive flesh.

This is what dieting is all about, trying to get rid of the uncomfortable cocoon that constricts us, depriving us of what we feel we deserve as human beings. It is about bringing out the image of us that we know people around us will appreciate. It is about reconciling our outer image with the inner image of the better self that we perceive as the authentic self, the self we identify with when we think of ourselves.

The importance of body images and the power of identification, often based on visual elements, did not go undetected in the work of Dr. Robert C. Atkins, one of many researchers and practitioners who have focused their efforts on all those who try hard to lose weight, often fighting against serious obesity and other weight-related problems, in order to improve their general health. Although Atkins never tackles the subject directly, passing references to body images and identification appear frequently in his writing. His most famous book, *Dr. Atkins' New Diet Revolution*, begins with these words: "Lose weight! Increase energy! Look great! This book will show you how it's done."[1]

In this chapter we will try to make sense of the connection between the Akins Diet plan and body identity. Reflection on the body and the embodied self is sparking growing interest not only among scholars and scientists but also in the media and popular culture. Hit TV shows such as *Extreme Makeover* or *The Biggest Loser* focus on the change of body images through plastic surgery, dieting, and extreme exercising. Other shows like *America's Next Top Model* and *Male Hunt* pursue ideals of beauty and success that actually embody commonly shared fantasies. The high ratings for these shows are a clear indication that those fantasies have a deeper and larger impact than we all would care to admit.

To get a better understanding of these phenomena, we will take up the analytical tools provided by a well-known yet controversial French psychoanalyst and theorist, Jacques Lacan.[2] Starting in the 1960s, this renowned intellectual tried to tackle some of these issues concerning body image and self-identity by developing a totally new practical approach and theoretical framework to psychoanalysis. Very provocative, not easy to read, and groundbreaking in many ways, Lacan has left a legacy that is still exerting a powerful influence, especially in Europe,

---

[1] Robert C. Atkins, *Dr. Atkins' New Diet Revolution* (New York: Avon, 2002), p. 3.

[2] For an introduction to Lacan's thought, see J. Scott Lee, *Jacques Lacan* (Amherst: University of Massachusetts Press, 1990).

where his ideas are being applied to cultural, social, and political issues.[3] We will refer in particular to what he labeled the "Imaginary" aspect of subjectivity, which can prove a very useful tool for analyzing the connections between images, culture, hunger, food, and desire.[4]

Before going any further, let's introduce a few key concepts that will us help understand the Lacanian take on inner life, culture, and desire.[5] First of all, let us tackle the Imaginary, the dimension of identification with visual images. Since childhood, we have learned to cope with a certain amount of confusion about ourselves. Who are we? How do we fit in the world that surrounds us? What is our role in the family in which we find ourselves? What are we supposed to do? These feelings generate constant insecurities, enhanced by the fact that, especially as infants, we do not have much control of our own bodies. We depend on others to be fed, to be cleaned, and to be protected. The images that surround us as infants and children, easily accessible and reassuringly undivided, provide us with the first safety net from those anxieties. As we will see, our own image as reflected from mirrors plays a key role in the development of our ego: looking at images, we learn to consider ourselves as individuals. According to Lacan, we construct the first core of our personality using external images, especially our own reflection, as building blocks. Nevertheless, these images are never neutral: they always come entangled in a network of meanings that are provided by our family, by the environment, by the culture in which we are born. The image of our body is never just the image of a body: in the eyes of the surrounding beholders—and as a consequence in ours—it is the image of a boy or of a girl, of a cute or of a not-so-cute child, of a good or of a bad child, of a son or a daughter, of a brother or a sister. These images introduce us to concepts and practices (age, sex, gender,

---

[3] See E. Laclau and C. Mouffe, *Hegemony and Socialist Strategy* (London: Verso, 1985).

[4] By subjectivity I indicate the subjective experience of self-conscious beings thats allow them to perceive themselves as autonomous individuals. See K. Silverman, *The Subject of Semiotics* (Oxford: Oxford University Press, 1983).

[5] For a more detailed introduction to Lacan's theories on desire, see Jacques Lacan, *The Four Fundamental Concepts of Psychoanalysis: The Seminar of Jacques Lacan*, Book XI (New York: Norton, 1981) and Slavoj Žižek, *The Ticklish Subject: The Absent Centre of Political Ontology* (London: Verso, 1999).

beauty, values, even desire) that make us functional members of a certain society, easing us into the roles that add another layer to our personality.

For Lacan this network of cultural and social elements, transmitted mainly by language, constitutes the "Symbolic," the second dimension of subjectivity. According to his theory, we are introduced into the Symbolic dimension as we learn how to understand and to use words, which can be considered symbols in that they stand for something else. In fact, words represent relationships, social structures, and cultural values that result from a collective attempt to make sense of the world that surrounds us. Nevertheless, this attempt is not always successful. There is always something that cannot be integrated in the symbolic network, something that keeps not making sense. For Lacan these disrupting elements constitute the "Real," the third dimension of the inner experience. The Real brings us back to our basic fears, to the unavoidable sense of mystery that surrounds us.[6] It reminds us that we do not have total control of ourselves, of our bodies, and of our surroundings. Recourse to an external authority (whose origin we do not understand but that we believe holds the power to give sense to reality) can be the solution to these anxieties.

In the case of diets, and Atkins in particular, this power belongs to science, as complicated and impenetrable as it seems. The scientist gives us all the answers we need. The less we understand the scientist's rationale, the easier it gets to make the leap of faith required to embark on a diet to change our body image.

We will see how some of Lacan's innovative concepts can throw an interesting light on the connections between food, desire, and pleasure in Dr. Atkins's work, and in the phenomenon of dieting in general.

Imaginary Bodies

Self-help literature is a thriving industry, responding to the needs of audiences always looking to progress in their lives, aiming at overcoming obstacles in their quasi-constitutionally-sanctioned pursuit of happiness. There is nothing wrong with

---

[6] See Slavoj Žižek, *Looking Awry* (Cambridge, Massachusetts: MIT Press, 1992).

it—most all of us strive to improve ourselves at all levels. We acknowledge that healthy self-esteem gives us better chances in our career, in our interaction with others, and in our emotional lives. When we appreciate ourselves, we unconsciously tend to send out positive vibes that the world around us seems ready to receive and reflect back to us. Our body language changes and communicates in different ways. It does feel good. In the first chapter of his book, Dr. Atkins actually gives us the visual picture of our future better self: "The you in the picture I'm conjuring up is finally the weight you've always had as your goal, or fairly close. You feel great—full of energy. Your skin is glowing with health. If you've been exercising, your toned muscles show it. The you in the picture isn't worried about weight loss anymore. You no longer need to spend your time planning the stages of a new diet, constantly concerned about your eating, feeling guilty when you break promises you've made to yourself" (Atkins, p. 5).

The mirror hovers in all diet books. Even when it is not directly mentioned, we are aware that it, together with the scale, is the first test dieters have to face to measure their improvements. In the case of Atkins, the image the mirror reflects clearly plays a major role in motivating dieting persons: every slight change, confirmed by the scale, gives them new reasons to hang in there and go through the Induction phase. On the other hand, body images, when they do not correspond to personal or social expectations, can also provoke frustration and anger. Dr. Atkins is aware of this danger, and he warns his readers about it. "You can make it the best body possible if you don't fall into the trap of demanding a perfect figure and weight loss schedule that exists only in your head" (Atkins, p. 281). And again, "building muscle mass does not mean becoming one of those bulging body builders. If you keep at it, you will begin to notice a gradual sculpting taking place under your skin—and I guarantee you're going to like how it looks" (Atkins, p. 293). The message is: use the improvements in your body image to gain courage to continue with the diet, but do not model the visual expectations with which you identify your inner self on images that are out of reach. We simply cannot attain a body type that is not ours. Rationally, we know it. Yet we are willing to incur great sacrifices to get as close as possible to those images, to the body types that we perceive as desirable.

The question is: where do these unrealistic images come from? Why do actors, models, body builders, and celebrities become so relevant in our fantasies? And why do they have such a power over us? If we abstract ourselves from all this for a second, we might start asking ourselves many questions. Who decided which body images are the right, successful, and positive ones? How does mainstream culture adopt these images? Or, rather, does mainstream culture create them? Why do these external and abstract images have such a strong clutch on our emotional well being? In general, why are images so important to our inner lives?

We can find some answers to these questions in Lacan's work. Based on his psychoanalytical experience, Jacques Lacan developed a theory that he defined as the "mirror stage." Analyzing dreams and recurring fixations of some patients, he realized how often images relating to the fragmentation of their body haunted them: limbs missing or misplaced, aggressive disintegration, the growth of wings. From where do these fears and anxieties come? He found the answer in the development of infants.

"The human child, at an age when he is for a short while, but for a while nevertheless, outdone by the chimpanzee in instrumental intelligence, can already recognize his own image as such in a mirror."[7] According to Lacan's observations, between six and eighteen months of age, infants are particularly taken with their own images as they see them reflected in mirrors. We all have enjoyed watching small babies playing in front of mirrors, making faces, discovering their own bodies and movements. Adults often join them in the games while holding them.

It is precisely to these games that Lacan imputes the relevance of body images for the human psyche. According to him, this intense interest is stimulated by the fact that the images reassure babies about the control they can actually exert over their own bodies, which they perceive as uncoordinated, out of control. After all, children cannot walk, many of their gestures and movements are tentative, and they cannot even feed themselves without the help of adults. The reflected images, on the other

---

[7] Jacques Lacan, "The Mirror Stage as Formative of the I Function," in *Ecrits: A Selection* (New York: Norton, 2002), p. 3.

hand, appear complete and co-ordinated in their actions. Lacan considers the children's condition as the consequence of a "veritable specific prematurity at birth" that traps their body in a "motor impotence and nursling dependence" (Lacan 2002, pp. 4–6).

The relief infants experience by looking at their own reflected images leads them to identify with them: the images are chosen as preferential selves, much more complete and self-sufficient than the ones experienced through their own developing bodies. The mirror image becomes the core around which the ego is constructed, an ego that is nevertheless ideal and external to the self.[8] It can be considered ideal in that is built around what we would like to be in order to respond to what the world around us considers us to be: good looking, strong, with our daddy's eyes. For this reason Lacan calls it the ideal-ego, functioning as a lighthouse in the building of a functioning individual.

This first identification process is at the same time reassuring but also alienating, since the ideal-ego is somehow fictional and located outside of the bodily self. Lacan ascribes to this element the frequent ambivalence that even as adults we all experience towards images or heroes or persons we identify with. We want to be like them, more or less consciously, but at the same time we hate them because we know we cannot be like them. In the case of Atkins's diet, the ideal-ego proposed as a stimulus to lose weight is what we want to look like and feel like. The ambivalence is lurking, right there: a slim figure is a goal that also scares us, because we fear that we might not reach it.

Atkins uses visualization to inspire his followers. The "you in the picture" is always there to provide resiliency to the dieting and often struggling self. After the Induction phase, where the Atkins neophyte is required to give up nearly all carbohydrates without renouncing other foods like protein and fat, "you are probably now catching glimpses of that new person on the horizon—if not in your own mirror. That new you is thinner, happier, healthier, and more confident" (Atkins, p. 154).

---

[8] "It suffices to understand the mirror stage in this context as an identification, in the full sense analysis gives to the term: namely, the transformation that takes place in the subject when he assumes an image—an image that is seemingly predestined to have an effect at this phase" (Lacan 2002, p. 4).

> Remember my suggestion to continually visualize yourself at your goal weight. Think about how much you deserve to look and feel good, to enjoy the happiness, health and sense of well-being that will come with your weight loss. (Atkins, p. 279)

In the Eye of the Beholder

Does this desire for a better body derive from the images themselves, or does it come from some other place? Even if the images—particularly their own reflections—provide children with protection and reassurance, they would appear to rely only on the visual elements that affect and shape the imaginary dimension. In themselves, images would not seem to be strong enough to exert such a great influence on the psyche. How can they become the base for the whole phenomenon of identification?

Growing up, we are offered other images to identify with by the surrounding social environment. In this case, though, we cannot forget that preferred body standards change with history and culture. In the Western world alone, for example, the Venus by Botticelli, a female character in a painting by Rubens, Marilyn Monroe, the 1970s fashion model Twiggy, and the more contemporary Jennifer Lopez embody very different ideals of female beauty. In contemporary U.S. culture, some ethnicities have clear preference for more sensual, voluptuous bodies. Context exerts a major influence, leading us to affirm that visual elements, without anchorage to something else, apparently do not have enough strength to activate a full-blown identification process. Without some cohesive thread, body images by themselves would be so fleeting that they would probably recreate the same anxieties and fears about dismemberment and lack of bodily control that they are supposed to exorcise in the first place.

Where does the power of the body images come from then? Does the identification work only at the level of the physical image or does it involve other elements? If we go back to the first imaginary identification of children with their reflected images, it's easy to realize that the relevance of those images as preferential ideals is not only motivated by their visual appeal. Other elements lead the child to identify with the reflected self. Think about how many times we have said to a child: how cute you are . . . how much you look like your mother . . . look at those lovely eyes . . . you're such a good girl . . . or well, let's hope the shape of that nose will change while growing . . . you remind me so much of that bastard of your father . . . what a bad girl you are! Many verbal elements interact to influence or reinforce the identification process that develops the core of the child's ego. The ideal-ego, based on the visual elements that children perceive of themselves in the mirror, are reinforced by what Lacan calls the ego-ideal, composed of all the elements that originate in other people's view of the child, their projections about her future, their take on what her personality should be. In this case, what counts is the perspective from which the child is viewed. The images reflected in the mirror, filtered through the gaze of family and friends, acquire meaning. The images become signs for something else. They come to stand for affection, family relationships, gender roles, and moral judgments. These cultural elements, deriving from the social, economic, and kinship structures of the community that incorporates the children, become part of the identification processes that shape the development of the child's ego.

Lacan defines this cultural network of meanings as the Symbolic, the second dimension of subjectivity. All of the elements of the definition stand for something else; hence they can be considered symbols. In Lacan's view, these symbols are not just juxtaposed, next to each other or piled up without any specific order: they constitute a system, where each element actually gets its meaning from its relationship with all the other elements composing the system. It is not so difficult as it sounds. Let's consider a few examples. You're in a restaurant and you need to go to the restroom. You will find two images on two doors: the silhouettes of a man and a woman. You will know which bathroom you are supposed to use because the two symbols are in opposition, incorporating the cultural difference in gender. In the case of a traffic light, a red light by itself would not mean much; it acquires its meaning in relation to a yellow and a green one. These observations will prove useful when we consider eating habits as a cultural system.

Besides responding to biological needs, food defines us as a society and as individuals. We could actually choose from a wide range of foods, but we usually limit our choices to the foods we have become used to since childhood, the food that defines our family and our culture. For example, in most of the

Western world larvae are not eaten, although they are eaten in other places and constitute a very effective source of nourishment. To take another example, foods are organized in dishes and the dishes in meals. Various meals are distributed during the day, during the week, and during the year, marking the different moments in time. If food is a cultural system, then, according to Lacan it cannot but be a part of the Symbolic. How does food specifically affect our relationship with our body images (the ideal-ego) and with the value that our culture grafts onto them (the ego-ideal)?

Dieting, not surprisingly, plays a key role. Let's go back to Dr. Atkins. We've seen how he employs body images to prod his followers to persevere in their dieting efforts. The body ideals to which Atkins refers are precisely those that are culturally perceived as more acceptable and, in some cases, desirable in our contemporary western societies: health, fitness, and slimness. The cultural and visual elements are tightly knit to create effective identification: by identifying with a specific body type, dieters not only satisfy their imaginary fantasies, but anchor themselves securely in the symbolic network of signs that constitutes their culture. The empty material body, made only of visual elements, fills up with meaning, as these visual elements become attached to this network of symbols.

We have seen how meanings in any culture constitute a system, where all the elements get their signification from their relations with all the other elements. We have also established that food is a cultural system. Within the food system, we can consider diets a specific subsystem, functioning according to interconnected rules and meanings. Dr. Atkins, it goes without saying, never forgets about food and eating habits, since the body constantly tells us that it needs nourishment. He clearly points out the direct connection between a negative body image and bad nutrition, which he considers a malfunctioning network (a cultural subsystem) of negative dietary practices, unhealthy food, and a generally defeatist attitude about food. At the same time, Atkins acknowledges the fact that insufficient food intake plays against achieving healthy nutrition patterns through dieting, and, as a consequence, can keep us from achieving the desired body image. "Deprivation is no fun. Once the biological gap between hunger and fulfillment grows too large, the rebound can be amazingly rapid as well as heartbreaking and humiliating. But that's the problem of diets that restrict quantities. The Atkins program refuses to accept hunger as a way of life"; "Nothing is more difficult to endure for a lifetime than being constantly hungry"; "Your resistance is at its greatest when you're satiated" (Atkins, pp. 10, 104, 247). The Atkins system perceives hunger as an uncontrollable instinct, a bodily necessity that surfaces when we least need it. In this sense, hunger definitely falls under the heading of "Real" in the Lacanian sense that we illustrated previously. It's something we can't control, something disrupting all our attempts at making sense of our body and its looks, but something with which we have to cope. Atkins often contrasts hunger with pleasure, which in his writing appears as something on which we have definitely more of a grip. "The controlled carbohydrate nutritional approach is not one of deprivation. Sheer hunger is the main reason for the failure of most weight loss efforts. A lifetime eating plan needs to be palatable, pleasant, and filling," and, "When doing Atkins, you'll find that your appetite has diminished, but your satisfaction from the food you eat has increased" (pp. 19, 44).

It is not only about counteracting the physical pangs of hunger. Dr. Atkins is well aware of the psychological relevance of food and of the satisfaction we derive from it. He affirms: "I equate healthy eating with gastronomic pleasure," "This is an obvious win-win situation. It offers you the pleasure of eating and the promise of being healthier than before" (pp. 5, 6). Dr. Atkins brings up contentment and fulfillment several times. "Eating Atkins-style is a food lover's dream come true—luxurious, healthy, and varied" (p. 19). "You're doing Atkins, and naturally you begin by eating—something you've previously done with some degree of guilt. Say good-bye to all that. It's time to plow into prime ribs and that cheese omelet" (p. 136). Dr. Atkins states: "I'll help you adopt a permanent way of eating that lets you lose weight without counting calories, makes you feel and look better, naturally re-energizes you, keeps lost pounds off forever with a lifetime nutritional approach that includes rich, delicious foods" (p. 4).

In Atkins's approach, not all victuals are necessarily evil. Only some specific elements of the food system are held responsible for our troubles. For this reason, we can successfully change our ways of eating, our habits, and to some extents our cultural tenets about what is good and bad for us without giving up pleasure and satisfaction. On the Atkins Diet you can still enjoy "rich, delicious foods."

Quilting the Flesh

What is the relation between hunger (the biological need for food), pleasure (the psychological state deriving from satisfying desire), body images, and the culture that provides and frames them in a wider context, making them more or less desirable?

In Lacan's theory the various elements in any system only acquire their meaning from each other and their mutual relations. In the case of food, for instance, breakfast acquires its own specific traits by being different from lunch and dinner. Within breakfast, cold cereals are opposed to oatmeal, croissants, and granola. When we choose one instead of the other, we give a certain character to our breakfast, and somehow we define ourselves, our eating habits, and the role that food plays in our culture. According to Lacan, though, these relations, and the role that each element plays in the system, are never stable. In the case of the American food system, for instance, lunch has lost much of its relevance over the past few decades, often ending up as just a snack on the go. The evening meal is no longer the center of the family life, but rather is often consumed by each member of the family at different times. Meaning, Lacan would say, is slippery and mutable, the result of continuous negotiations. The signs—the elements of the system—stay the same; it is their meaning that changes. In order for any cultural system to acquire a certain stability, allowing its users to share values, ideals, language, and the practices connected to them, certain signs must emerge as dominant, becoming the pivots around which all the other cultural signs determine and adapt their meanings. Lacan refers to these pivotal signs as "upholstering nails." The stuffing of a chair would go everywhere and create uncomfortable lumps if the nails in the upholstery did not keep it place. Likewise, meanings would shift constantly all over the place, staying undefined and confused, if some signs did not play the role of the nails, keeping the whole system in place.

If we analyze the food system in a given society, for instance, we notice how certain foods acquire more relevance, enjoying a symbolic weight that places them at the center of the social exchange that takes place around the table. In American society, foods such as the Thanksgiving turkey, hamburgers, barbecue, apple pie, Southern-fried chicken, and collard greens play a role in identifying a certain kind of diet.

Atkins is aware that the enticing body images that he projects to motivate his followers need anchoring in cultural, symbolic elements to acquire consistency and relevance. The upholstery nails in the food system he proposes are the "bad foods" that need to be avoided to reach the results we want: carbohydrates. Atkins's whole nutritional discourse revolves around them, in a neat and sensible way. "Those foods are bad for your health, bad for your energy level, bad for your mental state, bad for your figure. Bad for your career prospects, bad for your sex life, bad for your digestion, bad for your blood chemistry, bad for your heart. What I'm saying is that they are bad" (p. 15). Atkins frequently describes the excessive consumption of these foods, also called "trigger foods" (p. 219), as an addiction, or as an obsession, or even as enslavement (p. 139). When they give them up, dieters may even suffer from withdrawal symptoms "ranging from fatigue, faintness and palpitation to headache and cold sweats" (p. 141). More importantly, Atkins declares: "The most dangerous food additive on the planet is sugar in all its forms" (p. 253) and "Sugar is a metabolic poison" (p. 24). Sugar should not even be allowed to enter the dieter's home, for the benefit of the whole family (p. 253).

Around this main tenet, Dr. Atkins develops his entire scientific theory, reorganizing the whole field of nutrition and food-related health as we know it: carbohydrates are responsible for higher levels of insulin, diabetes, and high blood pressure. The need to avoid carbs revolutionizes one's food intake patterns, one's daily routine, and one's social life. Dieters' families are required to participate in their efforts to lose weight, while their friends are expected to accommodate their dietary needs. Such a profound change in culture and science reverberates through everyday life, in practices and common interactions. At a larger social level, interest in the Atkins Diet has given birth to a different lifestyle, leading to the creation of TV shows, various print-media publications, and the production and commercialization of new products, which sometimes entail the restructuring of the layout in retail stores and supermarkets.

A Leap of Faith

Atkins places carbohydrates, the "bad" elements that need to be avoided, at the center of his nutritional approach, reorganizing the dieting person's whole life and relationships with family and society. How is this possible? This lifetime commitment to the Atkins lifestyle requires a veritable act of faith, as Atkins himself repeatedly points out. "You must have faith," he proclaims, and later, "One of the obstacles you may find in the real world is people—the very same people upon whom you normally rely for advice and support" (pp. 136, 252). Those who do not follow Atkins are labeled as nonbelievers or naysayers (pp. 252–53).

The dedication of dieters to Atkins's plan clearly responds to a psychological need, otherwise the obedience and self-restraint the diet requires would not make sense. They would be too high a price to pay, if the reward were not substantial. What can this fundamental need be? Our body, since the infantile crisis that we solve by identifying with our own reflected image, is always a cause for puzzlement and a sense that we lack control. We can try as hard as we want, but we never fully understand the way our body grows, ages, and gains or loses weight. Our physical reality imposes itself over and over as something that does not always makes sense, despite all our attempts at rationalizations.

Our body never totally fits into the neat system of meanings that constitutes our culture, into the preferential images that we are offered, into the scientific knowledge that explains our biology. There's always too much fat, too many wrinkles, that annoying pain in the knee, the unexpected heart attack, or the anxiety we sometimes experience in front of food. "Your body has its own wisdom, so listen to it" (Atkins, p. 227). Atkins warns us: "Remember two things: First, your body is not a machine. Nor is it a duplicate of anyone else's body. It has its own system, its own agenda, and its own timetable. In the long run, it nearly always responds to sensible management by the person in charge—you. But, in the short run, your body may decide to go its own way, for its own reasons, which perhaps we don't understand. Don't get mad at it. It's a good body or it wouldn't have gotten you this far. Be patient; you can afford to outwait it" (p. 183). In statements such as these, Dr. Atkins portrays the body almost as something external, something that we cannot control, precisely when our most powerful and engaging fantasy consists of actually managing to gain control over it. The image of our slim body, which motivated us to start the diet in the first place, the experience of our body as something we can bend to our will, the received social values about beauty and attractiveness all gives way to the stubbornness of our unreasonable flesh.

Lacan defined the Real as all that subverts the expected order of the world that surrounds us, or at least our projections and hopes about it. According to Lacan, the Real is all that cannot be given a rational explanation, all that resists symbolization, in the sense that it cannot be absorbed in the network of meanings that our culture provides for us in order to make sense of our lives. Precisely for this reason, of course, the irruption of the Real into our internal reality is frightening. It reminds us of our frailty and of our inconsistencies. The symbolic and imaginary dimensions, on the other hand, offer respite from these fears, providing stable meanings, neat ideals, and confirmed practices. But at times these dimensions are not enough. We need to feel that our priorities and the meanings we give to reality are guaranteed by some external authority, something that gives them credibility and certainty. Since we cannot make sense of reality by ourselves, we need to believe that somebody knows its secret signification and is willing to bestow it on us, hence the need for all kinds of authorities organizing meanings in ways that make sense for us. In diets, "scientists" holds the authority to clarify an otherwise very confusing field of knowledge. They provide the upholstery nails that assure stability and certainty. In the case of Atkins the main "nail" is that carbs are bad. This is the organizing element that promises the return to a lost state of harmony, unity, and fullness, not only for our individual body but also for the community.[9] In this case, the fantasy is a food system and a market that works for the well-being and physical health of consumers, not just to sell and make money.

The presence of an external authority that guarantees meaning and good results also relieves the follower from decisions and choices. One is not to be blamed for desiring bad foods.

[8] Y. Stavrakakis, *Lacan and the Political* (London: Routledge, 1999), p. 52.

"Your compulsion holds no terrors," says Dr. Atkins. "Your food compulsion isn't a character disorder, it's a chemical disorder called hyperinsulinism" (Atkins, p. 44). "I am about to recount a horror story that might be headlined: Innocent Human is Turned Upon By Own Hormones!" (p. 53). "Let me explain something about cravings. . . . Your craving appeared, most likely, because it was triggered by a drop in your blood sugar" (p. 137). The uncontrollable body, or the frightening Real, to use the Lacanian terminology, is tamed by those bodily functions that play along the rules. "Lipolysis is one of life's charmed gifts. It's as delightful as sex and sunshine, and it has fewer drawbacks than either of them!" (p. 57).

So what is the dieter's role? On one side, embracing the certainty of the new lifestyle, there is no need for willpower: "Willpower is not the issue" (Atkins, p. 54). Dieters are repeatedly reassured about the fact that they will not be required to count calories, even when they find themselves busy counting carb grams. "I had too big an appetite and too little willpower, two facts that haven't changed much," admits Dr. Atkins (p. 61). "Superhuman willpower is not required to do Atkins, only the wisdom to put yourself into a position where you won't need it" (p. 140).

On one hand, Atkins frees overweight people from all moral accusations: "Part of the obesity epidemic we face in the United States may be due to the misconception that those of us who are overweight are simply gluttons or lazy couch potatoes" (p. 259). But then again, they get a warning: "Remember who's boss. You are absolutely in control of what goes in your mouth at all times" (p. 255).

"Internalize your responses to food so what used to be a struggle becomes a conscious choice, one that serves you for the rest of your life. . . . Learn how to deal with temptation. . . . Develop a style of eating for a lifetime" (p. 195). We detect a clear ambivalence: is the desire for bad food a fault of character or not? Dealing with the nightmare of carb gram counting, Atkins's voice becomes stern: "Counting grams of carbohydrate is truly your responsibility. If you don't count, you get in trouble" (p. 169). Also, calories reappear at times, for instance, when Atkins deals with exercise. "It's one of the basic laws of the universe: If you use more calories than you consume, you lose weight (You sharp-eyed readers might say, 'Whoa, I thought we didn't have to worry about calories!' That's true, but it's a great way, here, to illustrate an important point)" (p. 287). He explains, "Another way to organize your exercise is to count the calories you burn (You know I'm not going to ask you to count the calories you consume!)" (p. 291).

So although willpower is not deemed a key element in the diet, a certain degree of discipline is required. The body is disciplined and normalized not only regarding its food intake, but also in its inscription in a cultural system that gives it meaning, making it part of shared cultural practices. In the case of the Atkins Diet, the individual who desires to lose weight voluntarily adheres to a system of meaning that proposes a radical alternative to common perceptions of what is good and bad for your health, asks for a leap of faith, and gives easy, clear cut, and rational principles to follow. The body and its biological processes are given new, revolutionary meanings, all while being anchored to the common and popular ideals of physical beauty and health. By chosing a new point of reference, the danger of carbohydrates, Atkins shifts all the usual meanings and relocates them to create a system that offers an alternative to all those that have lost faith in other diets and in the possibility to acquire the body they desire. Filtered through the reassuring order of science and culture, the images they want to see reflected in the mirror can finally become flesh and blood.

16

Tyranny of the Carbohydrate: Feminist Dietary Drama

CORRINNE BEDECARRÉ

(Meeting in the café after the lecture on feminist pragmatism.)

DOROTHY: Marie, you look great. Are you on Atkins?

MARIE: No, I despise diets; I am a feminist.

DOROTHY: What does that have to do with feminism?

MARIE: Nothing. Atkins's diet and feminism go together like mustard and shoe polish. Will women ever spend their time on anything except their appearance? I can't go into a bookstore without seeing diet and cookbooks described as "self-help." The sheer number of people on the Atkins Diet alone is discouraging; and what a man's food fad it is, with meat, meat, meat, meat. But plenty of women are consumed with the minutiae of this Baroque diet. A person could learn Esperanto faster than the Atkins's "good carb" list. Just when it seems impossible to have diets become more ridiculous, Atkins comes out against non-starchy vegetables.

DOROTHY: I diet, I am a feminist, and I am not consumed with the minutiae of the regimen. I want my body to be lean and healthy. It is empowering for women to quit being passive about their health. Women of your generation did not understand their own bodies. The feminist manifesto of physical awareness, *Our Bodies, Ourselves*,[1] was revolutionary because

[1] Boston Women's Health Collective, *Our Bodies, Ourselves* (New York: Simon and Schuster, 1971).

it encouraged women to quit depending on the medical establishment and learn about their own bodies.

Marie: You evoke *Our Bodies, Ourselves* and yet take the bizarre advice of Dr. Atkins? He traded on his M.D. while trying to appear as the medical *outsider* giving "the people" the real story. Atkins is twenty-first-century snake oil. No reputable health organization unequivocally supports his methods as healthy. Women remain the primary food managers of our culture and many have uncritically accepted his highly debatable regimen.

Dorothy: But there is guarded acceptance by the health establishment of the effectiveness of Atkins's methods. Several studies are underway to compare longitudinal effects of various diet methods. Recently research has vindicated Atkins's supporters by dispelling the most serious worry of the diet: that it promoted heart disease. Followers have been shown to have reduced cholesterol and triglycerides, which is the gold standard for heart disease prevention. The knee-jerk criticism of anything new has been disproved: where are the predicted catastrophic massive heart attacks and kidney failure? They aren't happening.

Marie: Not yet.

Dorothy: Not yet? It has been around for four decades. But so much for the health report. I don't accept your charge that women are concerned with minutiae. Weight is trivial? Is everything concerned with our bodies trivial? The charge of appearance being only skin deep reflects latent dualistic holdovers. Descartes's assertion that humans are primarily and *essentially* thinking things accepts as human only our intellectual consciousness. He claimed our distinctive minds alone as human nature. Our physical consciousness he found of such inferior value that the body was defined as guided by instinct, not intelligence; passive, not active; and uncertain, not indubitable. For him, there is no knowledge in our sensing faculties and no logic to the signals and associations of the body. In our minds only we find the attributes shared with the divine: willfulness, intellection, and control. Our bodies partake of animal nature and therefore are subordinate and even functionally independent of our minds.

We haven't escaped this ideology. Every time people attend to their skin or muscles, they are "overly concerned" with their bodies. If they play memory games or solve math puzzles, they are improving them*selves*.

MARIE: And dieting transgresses dualism? That's ridiculous. Atkins talks about *controlling* one's body and rejecting its confused "addiction to carbohydrates." Our bodies are not to be trusted, according to the good doctor. They are prone to addiction of exactly those foods that do not lead to health. One must restrain and dominate the body. Atkins supports hierarchical dualism by pitting the superior mind against the unknowing, desiring body. The body doesn't know what's good for it.

Feminists have exposed Cartesian dualism for supporting sexism and racism. For Descartes, his thoughts *per se*—even if confused and deceptive—proved he was a *thinking* thing. But his bodily sensations, since illogical and unclear, did not in the same way prove he was an *embodied* thing. He *was* a mind, but he *had* a body. Since women are stereotypically defined by their bodies, their humanity has been dismissed. We are essentially too emotional, concrete, and changeable to support truth with a capital "T." Our so-called *essential* natures created conditions antithetical to the acquisition of knowledge. All people who worked with their bodies or were identified according to physical features were thought to be more aligned with animal nature. Atkins's approach is consistent with hierarchical dualism.

DOROTHY: You're being reactive without reflection. Look around you. Women have rejected dichotomous dualism and embraced their embodied selves. They believe they can be smart and fit, political and physical, lawyers and mothers, intellectual and beautiful. We embrace our embodiment; you try to ignore it.

A diet that explains the dynamics of the body and gives straightforward, effective advice for eating is not a tool of the master. It is a tool in any person's toolbox. Radical feminists bought the lie that being a mother was inherently oppressive. They did not want to be defined by their bodies so they silenced them. They did not want to be defined by societal standards of beauty so they claimed their autonomy by disregarding their appearance. That was reactive and in many ways capitulates to the dominating ethos. Isn't it just another way to be suspicious of the female form: hide it, deny it, and clearly don't reproduce because that is what women have been required to do?

Are Diets Women-Centered Projects or the Master's Tool?

MARIE: Feminism is not trying to tell women to stop having babies. Some of my best friends were babies. But child bearing has been a required function for women, often with few alternatives. Globally, when the education of girls rises so too does the age at which they bear children, and the number of females who choose not to have children. Those who do choose children have far fewer than before. Cross-culturally, when women have a choice they either do not want to be mothers or want their motherhood restricted.

DOROTHY: Women of color claim their motherhood as a hard won right!

MARIE: I agree that radical feminism can seem overly critical of some common women's projects, like motherhood. But how can dieting be liberatory? Women in our culture have unresolved relationships with their own bodies. I take issue with your tool analogy. Audre Lorde's great dictum: "The master's tools will never dismantle the master's house" fits here. The Atkins Diet is the master's tool.[2]

DOROTHY: Marie, female bodies are flourishing today. Look at Serena and Venus Williams: both of them are big, strong women and they are literally cover girls. Muscular, athletic, black sisters are tearing up the sports world. Title IX has created the first real generation of female athletes. They play

---

[2] Audre Lorde, "The Master's Tools Will Never Dismantle the Master's House," *Sister Outsider* (Freedom: Crossing Press, 1984), p. 110. Audre Lorde (1934–1992) described herself as "Black lesbian, mother, warrior, poet," and this was an understatement. She was one of the first theorists of color to challenge feminists about their roles in the academy and their own racism. Her insistence on truth-telling led her to articulate oppressive practices *within* feminist communities. Her article title demonstrates her rhetorical power.

hard, they understand sports, and they expect to be active, healthy, and physically competent. Atkins taps into that desire for energy and a strong body. We strongly value having a healthy body and we work at it. We don't glow; we sweat.

MARIE: Many women don't experience their bodies as forcefully athletic.

DOROTHY: I know what you mean. But that was truer twenty years ago. Iris Young's brilliant "Throwing Like a Girl" is difficult for some young women to understand.[3] Young observes movements of herself and other women as reflecting their subordinate status with space-conserving postures and limited motility. Her phenomenological[4] reading interprets women's hesitant movement as enacting internalized oppression. Obviously Young took as normative women whose class took them out of the realm of physical labor. Do some women today fear getting hurt and seeming too masculine? Sure. But many don't and we expect our bodies to be buff.

Women can claim their health and vitality with the Atkins Diet Revolution™. As Atkins says, "it's not really a diet; it's a way of life."[5] The lifestyle of healthy women comfortable in their own skin.

MARIE: Comfortable in their skin?!? I assume this is sarcastic. Women are rarely at ease with their bodies. Normal physical variations are experienced with shame, while self-hatred and starving are interpreted as mastery. Too many women share this *consuming* preoccupation with their bodies. The body is

---

[3] Iris Marion Young, *Throwing Like a Girl and Other Essays in Feminist Philosophy and Social Theory* (Bloomington: Indiana University Press, 1990), p. 148.

[4] The term "phenomenology" has been applied to the work of philosophers Husserl, Heidegger, and Merleau-Ponty. In response to philosophical traditions which focused upon discrete beliefs or perceptions, the phenomenologists considered the first-person experience more holistically. Consciousness is expanded past linguistic content of beliefs into the lived experience or conscious action.

[5] Robert C. Atkins, *Atkins For Life: The Complete Controlled Carb Program for Permanent Weight Loss and Good Health* (New York: St. Martin's Press, 2003), p. 26.

understood as the ultimate site of self-control. It's incredible to me that mainstream women are unable to achieve a critical consciousness about the massive efforts made to keep them focused on their bodies by idealizing unrealistic goals.

Mainstream women believe the hype about diet empowerment; it is all over the Atkins literature, websites, cookbooks, and blogs. Women "claiming back their lives" by *losing weight*! Do you realize, at the current rate, it will be a hundred years before women have political representation equivalent with their occurrence in the population? In the United States![6] Even if bodies are the chosen site of empowerment, there are more healthy orientations than dieting. Dieting is Empowerment Lite. How about accepting their skins with the Beyond Dieting™ program? Atkins keeps the focus on weight equilibrium as the zenith of personal achievement.

This is not new. Susan Bordo's wonderful *Unbearable Weight* is a sustained analysis of the terrible burden of women's own bodies.[7] Our society relentlessly subjects women to hypercritical scrutiny. When mainstream women finally break free of this self-loathing they will thank those, like Bordo, whose trenchant insights honor new visions of womanhood.

DOROTHY: Hey, Vagina Monologues, let me get a word in. You are being elitist and wrong about what losing weight means to women. Feminist philosophy is supposedly constrained by a rigorous commitment to taking the lives of actual women seriously. Yet, you want to disparage "mainstream women" without giving credit for their accomplishments. How do you think that Title IX translated from federal law to local-school actuality? Men and women all over the country have *demanded* sports opportunities for their daughters and they are getting them. At the last Olympics, one sports commen-

[6] Institute for Women's Policy Research, *Status of Women in the States* (Washington, DC: Institute for Women's Policy Research, 2004).

[7] Susan Bordo, *Unbearable Weight: Feminism, Western Culture, and the Body* (Berkeley: University of California Press, 1993). Bordo writes about subjectivity, embodiment, anorexia, and masculinity from a feminist perspective. Even those who do not agree with her conclusions will not easily refute her troubling analyses of contemporary female embodiment.

tator said the high profile of the female athletes was a direct result of their parents' and schools' massive support. The Society for Women in Philosophy has not been sponsoring soccer teams.

It is women in the trenches insisting on simple justice from their communities and from those they love who have forced the change. Women who have taken other paths are inspiration to women. But they are not doing the heavy lifting in the homes and schools all over the country.

MARIE: Dorothy, yes, female excellence in many fields is robust and growing, obviously. Yet, where are the other struggles for women's rights? Are women today *en masse* directing their efforts for the end of gender discrimination? I believe women have been resourceful in using their socially sanctioned roles as heterosexual wives and mothers to promote their daughters, which is important. But are they risking their relationships with men to advocate for their girls? Are the men's programs and the women's programs equivalent? Are the girls' teams coached by men? Are their daughters' rights to birth control and freedom from sexual violence being addressed? Isn't it easier to add teams than it is to train their sons to be sexually responsible and respectful?

DOROTHY: Women everywhere are asserting *their* needs and *their* desires. That's what feminism is about: providing equitable freedom for women. Feminism rejects women defined as male-helpmates and subordinates only. And it's happening. Dieting is a women's project. Low-carb has become a cultural mantra. Women have impacted the workplace, restaurants, and dining patterns and they are proving a force to be reckoned with.

Women can include weight management as a legitimate part of their experience of embodiment. They do not want to feel division between self and image. They want a unified experience. With Atkins they learn the process of creating ketosis to accelerate the metabolizing of stored fat. With Carb Counting Made Easy™, we can make our own decisions. It may sound funky but that is irrelevant. Are women doing what *they* want and accomplishing *their* goals by exercising and dieting? Yes!

Desiring Diet

Marie: But why do women want to diet? Let us return to Audre Lorde. She tells us, "The master's tools will never dismantle the master's house," and we need to meditate on that. Do you believe that you can empower yourself by playing right into the master's plan? The master's house of inequality shouldn't be retrofitted with tampons to accommodate women. It's a house built on inequality and domination. It rests its foundation on the backs of others. We need to understand how dieting supports domination—not claim it as our own tool. Women's bodies have been under male control long enough. We should not take their preoccupation with our bodies as our own preoccupation.

Dorothy: You have me a little worried here. Weight *can* be unbearable. Our culture is seriously endangered by obesity.

Marie: I think there's reason to be worried. Consider women's monitoring of their own and other's weight. Compare it to some objectively serious information. You can remember the body form of hundreds of women you know. You can remember if their weight was "up" or "down" at different times of their lives. What about their debt load, the interesting projects of their lives, or whether they were paid as much as their co-workers? Why do we know what we know? It is more than just the difference between visible and invisible. Our attention indicates priorities and the priorities are not in our interests—so how are they "our" priorities?

The most effective form of control is reinforced internally. Men don't have to objectify us alone, because we are happy to help out.

Dorothy: Claiming my body is not the same as objectifying it. I want a fit, toned body.

Marie: The perfect sleight of hand. The real meat of your life is your meatiness. Women do not frequently discuss money matters that affect their lives extensively. Women discuss food and diets and their bodies. Atkins provides a brilliantly consuming model to follow. Come on, ladies, follow the steps, the sequences, the lists and *take control of your life.* Don't bother with justice or equality or solidarity—time to trim that waist.

DOROTHY: Marie, how do you sleep at night? There is no diet conspiracy to keep women out of the Senate. Atkins has steps, of course. It is organized and systematic. Life is very complicated and women's lives especially so. Who cares if Atkins is programmatic? That is a strength, not a weakness.

Women notice each other's weight and talk about food because food is important. It is sexist to revile "women's work" in the kitchen as female servitude. Food is culture and love and pleasure.

MARIE: I want to reach you on this. I never said cooking or eating was the problem. Dieting and focusing on twenty pounds to the detriment of focusing on gender inequality in health care is the problem. In the twentieth century someone observed women should raise more hell and fewer dahlias. In this century women should stop dieting and start living. There is no conspiracy to make women obsessively focus on their figures. As Foucault[8] writes, modern power is characterized by being decentralized and internalized. We have *become* a surveillance society, and we monitor ourselves and others to maintain social order as defined by those in power. No single agency need exert dominating control as *all* members and entities monitor and reinforce the status quo.

Our bodies are political. *Everyone* will notice when someone loses weight and is told they look fabulous. *We* internalize tension when we teeter above the ridiculous standards of emaciated models. Foucault's model fits with the diet preoccupation in general and Atkins in particular. Women are to be pretty, women are to look nice, and this means look thin. Forget the secret diet police: every mirror becomes a guard, every scale an alarm.[9]

DOROTHY: Even if I did agree with you on this point, this doesn't prove that dieting can't be a good temporary tool for health. People are not anywhere near model-thin in the United

---

8 Michel Foucault (1926–1984) was a French philosopher who wrote about the relationship between power and knowledge. In his work on prisons, especially, he looks at ways in which society trains the body ideologically and physically.

9 Michel Foucault, *Discipline and Punish* (New York: Vintage 1979); *The History of Sexuality, Volume 1: An Introduction* (New York: Vintage, 1980). As cited in Bordo, *Unbearable Weight*, p. 302.

States. We are fat and getting fatter. We might have to do what is necessary to get to a healthy place and then we can fight bigger battles.

MARIE: The Atkins Diet is never over. It begins with the ominously named Induction Cycle™ designed to break the stranglehold of carbohydrate addiction. This cult model of indoctrination requires dramatic elimination of carbohydrates to produce an atypical metabolic process called ketosis. This is followed by the Ongoing Weight Loss™ cycle in which *five grams* of carbohydrates a *week* are added. With increments like this, what else could anyone do?

DOROTHY: Any major habit changes will take attention.

MARIE: It is beyond attention. The first intense phases are followed by more self-surveillance. Moreover we are celebrated when we demonstrate our domination of our bodies. We receive positive attention and feel good about ourselves. Then Pre-maintenance™ is followed by Lifetime Maintenance™. Most dieters never get to this level. Most dieters keep cycling through early stages, which are characterized by quick weight loss and returning to old habits. But even *ideally*, an Atkins dieter remains on Lifetime Maintenance™. Monitoring, watching, and controlling one's behavior through constant attention. Even Foucault couldn't have imagined this maniacal level of hyper-vigilance.

DOROTHY: You make this sound evil. The dieter *wants* to lose weight. When they have their ACE™ (Atkins Carbohydrate Equilibrium™) they will then be in control of their weight. Many reputable sources on weight loss agree that by attending to what one eats consumption will be reduced.

MARIE: The standard for attention is food diaries. This simple non-trademarked method helps one to notice food patterns and to create incentive for not snacking throughout the day. The number one reason that people lose weight is they eat fewer calories than they use. Calories are virtually invisible in the Atkins system. He gives the impression that as long as a person is eating the "right foods" they will lose weight. The AGR™ (Atkins Glycemic Ranking™) and ANA™ (Atkins Nutritional Approach) focus attention, yes, but they also focus attention on themselves. Desire again is created for something different than what is actually needed. You don't *need* to know the AR™ (Atkins Ratio), which compares antioxidant capacity to grams of carbs. Most people in the world wouldn't know an antioxidant from the Antichrist and they are not obese.

DOROTHY: We can't fight feminist battles if we are fighting our bodies.

MARIE: Now we are in agreement. We need to enjoy our bodies and feel accepting of their bulges and curves. Food is one of life's great pleasures. Yet women are told to restrict their enjoyment and parse their pleasure. I am really on a Bordo kick today, but her work comparing advertising of women and men's relationships to food, is amazing. We learn "how to handle a hungry man" with big meaty servings while women "indulge" in miniscule containers of low-fat yogurt. The shame of being an out-of-control woman is a constant theme in diet ads. Feminists want to enjoy their bodies and their animal nature. Let's be embodied as we really are and let out the waistband. How does Atkins support that?

DOROTHY: Atkins has been called the hedonistic diet because it gives people protein and substantial foods that are satisfying. Starvation is not Atkins. Why do you think it is so popular? People can eat and lose weight. We teach our bodies to desire what they need. It encourages cheese, butter, meat, and berries. It retrains eating to be filling but nutritious. It gives control back to you.

Tyranny of the Carbohydrate

MARIE: And what are you to control? Carbohydrates. We are alleged to be addicted to carbohydrates. How can women break through the substantial barriers of millennia-old gender oppression if we are on Lifetime Maintenance™? We must remain vigilant against encroaching, insidious weight. The weight is our personal problem. It is up to us. Women are to resist the putative tyrannical forces of carbohydrates.

DOROTHY: But surely the American diet is roundly criticized for unhealthy foods. That's not Atkins's problem. Atkins gives us tools to better understand our bodies and our metabolism. This is the soul of empowerment: gaining knowledge, making choices, achieving goals. I am woman, hear me roar.

Marie: You mean, hear you rare. Bears don't eat that much meat. What are the great tools of Atkins? Atkins reiterates the cliché that "empty calories are empty"—that is not a significant addition to the corpus of diet lore.

Yes: reducing carbs can help one lose weight. Here is the misdirection: Atkins obscures true social causes and emphasizes personal responsibility. Obesity as a widespread phenomenon and dieting as a social practice are direct results of sprawling industrialization. We drive between suburbs without city centers to workplaces without physical activity. The relative affluence and super-sized packaging of food have more than doubled serving sizes since the 1970s. This has led to substantial weight gain, even in children.

The true causes of obesity are not individual; they are social and cultural. People are socially constructed, and the body functions *culturally* as well as *physically*. The effects of various cultural choices are inscribed and embodied in the forms of their populace. Due to development with cars and not people in mind, we are the heaviest population in the world, but other industrialized nations are catching up.

Dorothy: But this is our life. We deal.

Marie: But why are we getting fat? Why? According to Atkins it is because of empty calories, inappropriate addictions. But according to global trends, fat is a byproduct of our cultural choices. People's weight gains correlate with sprawl, with lack of exercise, with detachment from food production. The feminists' mantra is "The Personal is Political." Your personal struggle with fat is not just about *you alone*, it is about *you as an American*.

Let us quit pointing at the fat kid and build pedestrian-friendly neighborhoods. Our demon is not the insidious baguette but our collective decisions that ultimately corrode our quality of life, our humanness, and also make us fat.

Dorothy: Okay. I want to live in the Renaissance village, too. But in the meantime, we must accept our suburban realities. We're bigger than is healthy and we need an effective method for controlling our weight. Atkins Quick Quisine™ gives us that.

Marie: Have you noticed I mentioned no physiological processes in the causes of obesity? This is not, by the way, a feminist description. Multiple sources like the National Weight Control Registry, the Federal Trade Commission, and the American Obesity Association cite these findings. When a woman's probability of obesity can be determined by her geographic location, distance from a metropolitan area, ethnic group, socioeconomic class, and occupation, how can it be blamed on the Dreaded Addictive Carbohydrate (TM pending)?

Atkins talks about personal choices, not social forces, and in doing so addresses a relatively minor variable. Do you really believe women in Ghana have less carbohydrate addiction than women in the U.S.A.? Or Egypt? Or Costa Rica?

Dorothy: So what? What can I do? Atkins is not denying the social conditions of modern life. The only thing I have control over is what I put in my mouth. Even existentialists do not dispute the "facticity" of one's life.[10] Yes, there are material constraints, but they have an elastic nature and do not in and of themselves determine the outcome; they just constrain certain choices. We are in bad faith when we abdicate our lives and believe we are not in control. No one has perfect control; everyone has limitations and constraints on the facts of their lives. Atkins exhorts us to claim responsibility for our lives.

Marie: You life is not your carb count. People are claiming responsibility for more than they should. And we are not taking responsibility for changing our circumstances. You're the one who doesn't believe in conspiracies and yet you think *they* control our communities? We can change our communities. But we'll never demand and create different communities if we identify the problem as too many donuts.

Don't Get Me Started

Dorothy: Modern women do not want to look to urban sprawl or capitalism or Christianity to rule their lives. They claim their lives and are working it. We run, we climb, we canoe,

---

[10] Existentialists use the word "facticity" to refer to unchangeable factors in one's life. For example, a birthplace. It mimics "plasticity" in that although one's birthplace may be determined, one's response to one's birthplace is not.

and we do yoga. We claim our own ideas about our desired forms. Some popular female forms are brutally thin—I will admit that. But the other dominant female form is athletic and buff. Look at the arms of those actors at the Academy Awards. One woman after another strode confidently to the podium with arms that were cut. They were not starved into those outfits; they earned those looks. The new paradigm is someone who is flexible, strong, well-defined, and easy in her own skin.

MARIE: Now that latte is causing you to hallucinate. The new model leaves no part of her natural. She fake bakes, she has her nails done, her eyebrows waxed, her hair dyed, and her pubic hair eliminated. And still she gets airbrushed. She may not want to be a little girl but she definitely wants to look plastique. She is as afraid of her body as was Descartes.

DOROTHY: Okay, now we are on. You are part of the second wave and this is third wave feminism we are talking about.[11] We don't buy some of your most treasured claims. The real woman does not have to be ugly. We don't intend to be Earth Mothers or Mary Daly Hags. We do not fear our cyborg, augmented "nature." Pacemakers, in-vitro fertilization, contact lenses, birth control medication implants, artificial knees, antidepressants, dental fillings: bring it on and make us better. More tools. Human nature is malleable, female nature is malleable, and we are pushing the limits.

MARIE: But do your models transgress the status quo? Do they challenge the borders of female domination or do they just update the female stereotype? A Brazilian wax is just the latest way to sexualize childhood and to express disgust in adult womanly bodies. Women "want" exaggerated breast

[11] American feminists claim three waves of modern feminism. The nineteenth-century suffragists began the struggle with the fight for political representations. Mid-twentieth century, 1970s, feminists are known as "second wave" feminists. This is still a vital feminist force and has been dominated by questions regarding locations of oppression and intersecting forms of oppression such as class and gender. By the 1990s, young feminists were claiming a "third wave" of feminism. These women have grown up with the benefits hard-won by second wavers. Feminism, despite popular mythology, has always had an irreverently funny bent. Nevertheless, third wavers have a pronounced playful, sassy aspect evidenced by *Bitch* magazine and Grrrl blogs.

implants combined with a pre-adolescent pubic area. That is shocking to feminists who question the incessant requirements of women to be visually appealing by suppressing their natural forms.

Dorothy: I might agree with you about the Brazilian wax, but I might not. You have too many rules for what a feminist should look like. What is the virtue of being ugly for ugliness' sake?

Marie: You continue to equate "natural" with "ugly." Your words, not mine. No one is requiring a feminist uniform. We explicitly support a plurality of bodies. The status quo wants to make everyone blonde and without blemishes—while defining virtually everything as a blemish.

Dorothy: Are you sure we are not trapped in the Sixties mindset?

Marie: It is naive to disregard the intense efforts to domesticate women. Look at how society reacts to any alternative to heterosexuality for women. Lesbians and bisexual women embody the female form that is not solely available for male pleasure. The culture is uncomfortable with women escaping stereotypic definition. Notice how often independent women supporting women-centered projects are called "lesbians" as if this is a criticism. Women who dress and live for themselves or other women are "manly" and challenged as being full of testosterone. On the other hand, society is titillated by renegade behavior. Female-centered sexuality has been coopted as an object of male pleasure.

You act as if the work is over. Old battles are over. Women can wear pants. But are there new ways to control and limit women? Of course, and dieting is as good as it gets.

Dorothy: Some timid females afraid of their husbands' disapproval might diet. But dieting is not intrinsically dominating. Obesity shortens women's lives. Fat is not a myth. Fat is a reality and is getting more real all the time. Fat is a live issue right now.

Marie: I am worried that you are too complacent about the need for women to beautify. Feminists need to be attentive to the insidious forms of social control that, when internalized, feel as if they are self-generated, not imposed from without.

DOROTHY: Look at your female ideals compared to mine. Here in my copy of *Willful Virgin*, Marilyn Frye[12] describes her imaginative construction of the Willful Virgin as a wild, undomesticated female creating herself. I am good with that. And when she goes on to claim, "these Virgins do not attire and decorate themselves in the gear which in their cultures signal female compliance with male-defined femininity and which would form their bodies to such compliance," I am still down with that. Obviously women control their appearance.

But then Frye says that Willful Virgins "do not make themselves 'attractive' in the conventional feminine modes of their cultures and so people who can ignore their animal beauty say they are ugly."[13] Here is my question: Must contemporary feminists accept Frye's rally for righteous ugliness?

MARIE: Yes and no. Women claim their wild beauty and maybe some will find women too wild to be beautiful. That is their problem.

DOROTHY: But ugliness is a *virtue* for some feminists. It's considered a transgressive accomplishment. A woman shouldn't "have" to be beautiful, especially in a conventional sense, to be respected or to be considered womanly. But ugly? Ugly happens. But it is not *de facto* feminist.

MARIE: This is an important disagreement. Women must be separated from their appearance, culturally. It is sexist to burden women with beauty. Men do not bear this burden. They are valued as interesting or manly even if fairly unattractive, not to mention fat.

DOROTHY: We are not burdened with conventional "beauty." Tattoos and piercing are considered edgy and beautiful. We use our bodies as canvasses. We do not dress up for men: we dress up for ourselves. We don't have to wear pants or skirts. We can wear pants and skirts. Go to a college classroom and

---

[12] Marilyn Frye is a founding mother of the Society of Women in Philosophy, Midwest Division. She teaches at Michigan State, Lansing. Frye's *Politics of Reality* is widely used in women's studies and philosophy courses. An analytically trained philosopher, she combines unflinching feminist critique with clarity and creativity. Many of her essays are found in philosophy anthologies.

[13] Marilyn Frye, *Willful Virgin: Essays in Feminism 1976–1992* (Freedom: Crossing Press, 1992), p. 134.

see if the men and the women are all gender-bending like crazy. Men have pink hair and t-shirts with cartoons while women have spikes in their eyebrows and shaved heads. The standards for dress and movement for men and women have changed and feminism needs to respond to that change. No more Madonna-whore dichotomies. We go Boho, skater, hip hop, Euro trash, diva, Goth, nerd, techno, punk, jock—whatever. We even admire big women who make it work.

Marie: We applaud the originality and edginess of Grrrl feminism. But it's premature to be claiming victory. We want full-blooded emancipated embodiment. The diet industry typified by the mega-corporate Atkins Diet™ can only lead to embodiment lite.

Dorothy: Would this be a bad time to bring up the French women's diet?

The Low-Carb Canon

The health and diet section of any American bookstore is packed with a huge variety of low-carb diet books. To help you separate the burger from the bun, here's our list of superstars: the most influential, popular, and important diets to date in the low-carb *oeuvre.*

Agatston, Arthur, M.D. *The South Beach Diet: The Delicious, Doctor-Designed, Foolproof Plan for Fast and Healthy Weight Loss.* New York: St. Martin's, 2005. (Hardback published by Rodale in 2003.)

Dr. Agatston's book begins with the declaration, "The South Beach Diet is not low-carb." Yet its initial two-week phase disallows all bread products, rice, potatoes, pasta, fruit, sugar, and alcohol. Thereafter, the dieter can eat modest amounts of carbohydrate foods chosen from the low end of the glycemic index. Agatston, a cardiologist, gives a thorough explanation of how overconsumption of quick-digesting carb foods, such as white bread, can foster diabetes, heart disease, and weight gain. This diet doesn't require any counting of carbs or calories, but it does ask the dieter to choose healthy oils and avoid saturated fats. Has recipes from tony Miami-area restaurants.

http://www.southbeachdiet.com/

Atkins, Robert C., M.D. *Dr. Atkins' New Diet Revolution.* New York: Avon, 2002.

The granddaddy of all low-carb diets, Dr. Atkins's book has the strictest carb limitations, the most gripping prose, incredible longevity (it first appeared over thirty years ago), and arguably the most complete scholarly documentation for scientific claims. Atkins sings the praises of ketosis (a.k.a. lipolyosis, a process in which your body uses fat stores for fuel), which he explains in nontechnical language. Highly persuasive, and chock full of practical tips for eating low carb in a junk food world.

http://atkins.com/

———. *Atkins for Life*. New York: St. Martin's, 2003.

Atkins for Life is for seasoned Atkins dieters who have enjoyed success on the program. Has advice about how to find a level of carb consumption appropriate for maintaining weight, many recipes and meal plans, and personal stories of Atkins dieters.

Audette, Ray, with Troy Gilchrist. *NeanderThin: Eat Like a Caveman to Achieve a Lean, Strong, Healthy Body*. New York: St. Martin's, 1999.

The key to the NeanderThin diet is to imagine that you have no technology available to you except a sharp stick or rock, and to eat only the foods attainable under those circumstances. Thus, you may eat as much meat, fish, fruit, vegetables, nuts, seeds, and berries as you like (the author does recommend cooking your meat, to avoid food poisoning). Grains, beans, potatoes, dairy products, and sugar are verboten. Audette, a falconer by profession, claims that the result is unprecedented good health as well as weight loss.

http://www.neanderthin.com/

Cordain, Loren, Ph.D. *The Paleo Diet: Lose Weight and Get Healthy by Eating the Food You Were Designed to Eat*. Hoboken: Wiley, 2002.

Cordain presents the Paleo Diet as different from and superior to "fad low-carb diets," which he roundly criticizes. The Paleo Diet features large quantities of lean meat, fruits, and nonstarchy vegetables, and moderate quantities of nuts and seeds. It prohibits the following: dairy products; cereals in any form; legumes; salty, fatty, or processed meats; and all other processed foods. This diet is potentially much higher in carbs than Atkins, as the dieter can eat unlimited amounts of fresh fruit. It strictly limits salt and "bad" fats (saturated fat, trans fat) and focuses on the "acid-base imbalance" of the American diet: we eat too many acid-forming foods such as grains and dairy, and too few alkaline-forming fruits and vegetables, with myriad health consequences.

http://www.thepaleodiet.com/

Eades, Michael R., M.D., and Mary Dan Eades, M.D. *Protein Power.* New York: Bantam, 1996.

The Eadeses' book is ideal for those who want to know all about the science behind low-carb dieting. The authors explain the body's insulin-glucagon system in readable detail, and give mathematical formulas for calculating ideal weight, body mass index, body fat percentage, and lean body mass. This diet pays more attention to protein than Atkins does; central to the program is calculating protein needs based on your lean body mass and being sure to consume that amount each day. Its carb allowances are a bit more liberal than Atkins's, but it requires counting carbs *and* counting grams of protein consumed.

http://www.eatprotein.com/

Rubin, Jordan. *The Maker's Diet: The 40-Day Health Experiment that Will Change Your Life Forever.* Lake Mary: Siloam, 2004.

A bestseller in the "Christian weight loss" category, the Maker's Diet requires dieters to give up nearly all carbs in the first stage of dieting; carbohydrate intake is limited thereafter. Taking a faith-based rather than a science-based approach, it is ostensibly modeled after the diet of biblical peoples and ritually forbids certain foods, such as pork and shellfish, in addition to all highly processed foods. Contains other prescriptions with biblical origins, about, for instance, hygiene and prayer.

Sears, Barry. *The Zone: A Dietary Road Map.* New York: ReganBooks, 1995.

A decade old, the Zone diet remains tremendously popular to this day. The program involves carefully balancing protein, fat, and carbohydrate consumption in the proportion of 30/30/40.

This ratio is considerably lower in carbs and higher in protein and fat than the typical American diet. Carbs low on the glycemic index, small meals, exercise, and healthy fats are other important parts of the diet. As *Protein Power* does, the Zone requires calculating individual protein requirements based on lean body mass. Contains a wealth of medical detail, including one of the first popular expositions of eicosanoids (intracellular hormones), which, according to Sears, profoundly influence health and happiness, and are kept in proper balance by the Zone diet.

http://www.zonediet.com/

Philosophy and Food: Some Gleanings

If you're interested in continuing to explore food in a philosophical way, here are some books to get you started.[1] A warning: the historical texts may contain relatively little direct discussion of food; you may have to read between the buffet lines to find the meat of the issue. (We've quoted some passages from them, to start you salivating.) The contemporary works, on the other hand, are among the small but growing list of works that explicitly identify food as their primary topic. Philosophers, it seems, are beginning to talk with our mouths full.

Old Country Buffet

ARISTOTLE. *De Anima.* Translated by J.A. Smith. Pelagus website, http://www.pelagus.org/books/ON_THE_SOUL,_by_Aristote_1.html.

Since nothing except what is alive can be fed, what is fed is the besouled body and just because it has soul in it. Hence food is essentially related to what has soul in it. Food has a power which is other than the power to increase the bulk of

[1] Thanks to Ken Albala, Tom Alexander, Ray Boisvert, Jeremy Iggers, Glenn Kuehn, and Fabio Parasecoli for their contributions to this list of works. Most of the historical works are available in many editions and multiple translations, both in paper and on the internet. We've included bibliographic information for the versions from which the quotations are taken. There is nothing sacred about these versions.

what is fed by it; so far forth as what has soul in it is a quantum, food may increase its quantity, but it is only so far as what has soul in it is a 'this-somewhat' or substance that food acts as food; in that case it maintains the being of what is fed, and that continues to be what it is so long as the process of nutrition continues.

ARISTOTLE. *Ethics.* Translated by W. D. Ross. Pelagus website, http://www.pelagus.org/books/NICOMACHEAN_ETHICS,_by_Aristotle_1.html.

In everything that is continuous and divisible it is possible to take more, less, or an equal amount, and that either in terms of the thing itself or relatively to us; and the equal is an intermediate between excess and defect. By the intermediate in the object I mean that which is equidistant from each of the extremes, which is one and the same for all men; by the intermediate relatively to us that which is neither too much nor too little—and this is not one, nor the same for all. For instance, if ten is many and two is few, six is the intermediate, taken in terms of the object; for it exceeds and is exceeded by an equal amount; this is intermediate according to arithmetical proportion. But the intermediate relatively to us is not to be taken so; if ten pounds are too much for a particular person to eat and two too little, it does not follow that the trainer will order six pounds; for this also is perhaps too much for the person who is to take it, or too little—too little for Milo, too much for the beginner in athletic exercises. The same is true of running and wrestling. Thus a master of any art avoids excess and defect, but seeks the intermediate and chooses this—the intermediate not in the object but relatively to us.

Like Aristotle? Perhaps you'll also like . . .

"The Aristotle Diet." *Fides Quaerens Intellectum: An Exploration of Culture, Politics, and Philosophy through the Eyes of a Philosophy Graduate Student, Or Just a Place for Me to Vent,* http://blog.johndepoe.com/2004/08/aristotle-diet.html.

The diet inspired by the philosopher!

BRILLAT-SAVARIN, ANTHELME. *The Physiology of Taste.* Translated by Fayette Robinson. The University of Adelaide Library website, eBooks@Adelaide, http://etext.library.adelaide.edu.au/b/brillat/savarin/b85p/

AN IMMENSE OBESE.—Do me the favor to pass me the potatoes before you. They go so fast that I fear I shall not be in time.

I.—There they are, sir.

OBESE.—But you will take some? There are enough for two, and after us the deluge.

I.—Not I. I look on the potato as a great preservative against famine; nothing, however, seems to me so pre-eminently to fade.

OBESE.—That is a gastronomical heresy. Nothing is better than the potato; I eat them in every way.

DOGEN AND KOSHO UCHIYAMA. *From the Zen Kitchen to Enlightenment: Refining Your Life.* New York: Weatherhill, 1983.

We are, therefore, the personification of the universe when we eat—this is a fact that only the Buddhas fully understand—and the universe is the personification of Truth. When we eat, the universe is the whole Truth in its appearance, nature, substance, force, activity, cause, effect, relatedness, consequence and individuality. The Truth manifests itself when we eat and, when eating, we can realize the manifestation of Truth. The correct mind, when eating, has been Transmitted from one Buddha to another and creates ecstasy of both body and mind. (from "Meal-time Regulations")

EPICURUS. Letter to Menoeceus. Translated by R. D. Hicks. Masachusetts Institute of Technology website, the Internet Classics Archive, http://classics.mit.edu/Epicurus/menoec.html.

Again, we regard independence of outward things as a great good, not so as in all cases to use little, but so as to be contented with little if we have not much, being honestly persuaded that they have the sweetest enjoyment of luxury who stand least in need of it, and that whatever is natural is easily procured and only the vain and worthless hard to win. Plain fare gives as much pleasure as a costly diet, when once the pain of want has been removed, while bread and water con-

fer the highest possible pleasure when they are brought to hungry lips. To habituate one's self, therefore, to simple and inexpensive diet supplies all that is needful for health, and enables a man to meet the necessary requirements of life without shrinking, and it places us in a better condition when we approach at intervals a costly fare and renders us fearless of fortune.

HIPPOCRATES. *On Ancient Medicine.* Translated by Francis Adams. Masachusetts Institute of Technology website, the Internet Classics Archive, http://classics.mit.edu/Hippocrates/ancimed.html.

Let your food be your first medicine.

HUME, DAVID. "Of the Standard of Taste." Theodore Gracyk's Home Page (personal home page), Minnesota State University Moorhead, http://www.mnstate.edu/gracyk/courses/phil%20of%20art/hume%20on%20taste.htm.

It is acknowledged to be the perfection of every sense or faculty, to perceive with exactness its most minute objects, and allow nothing to escape its notice and observation. The smaller the objects are, which become sensible to the eye, the finer is that organ, and the more elaborate its make and composition. A good palate is not tried by strong flavours; but by a mixture of small ingredients, where we are still sensible of each part, notwithstanding its minuteness and its confusion with the rest. In like manner, a quick and acute perception of beauty and deformity must be the perfection of our mental taste; nor can a man be satisfied with himself while he suspects, that any excellence or blemish in a discourse has passed him unobserved. In this case, the perfection of the man, and the perfection of the sense or feeling, are found to be united. A very delicate palate, on many occasions, may be a great inconvenience both to a man himself and to his friends: But a delicate taste of wit or beauty must always be a desirable quality; because it is the source of all the finest and most innocent enjoyments, of which human nature is susceptible.

KANT, IMMANUEL. *Critique of Judgment.* Translated by James Creed Meredith. Pelagus website, http://www.pelagus.org/books/THE_CRITIQUE_OF_JUDGEMENT,_by_Immanuel_Kant_1.html.

So far as the interest of inclination in the case of the agreeable goes, every one says "Hunger is the best sauce; and people with a healthy appetite relish everything, so long as it is something they can eat." Such delight, consequently, gives no indication of taste having anything to say to the choice. Only when men have got all they want can we tell who among the crowd has taste or not.

KIERKEGAARD, SØREN. "In Vino Veritas." Part 1 of *Stages On Life's Way*. Christian Classics Ethereal Library website, http://www.ccel.org/k/kierkegaard/selections/veritas.htm.

[Victor Eremita speaks:] **Now I demand the greatest superabundance of everything thinkable. That is, even though everything be not actually there, yet the possibility of having it must be at one's immediate beck and call, aye, hover temptingly over the table, more seductive even than the actual sight of it. I beg to be excused, however, from banqueting on sulphur-matches or on a piece of sugar which all are to suck in turn. My demands for such a banquet will, on the contrary, be difficult to satisfy; for the feast itself must be calculated to arouse and incite that unmentionable longing which each worthy participant is to bring with him. I require that the earth's fertility be at our service, as though everything sprouted forth at the very moment the desire for it was born. I desire a more luxurious abundance of wine than when Mephistopheles needed but to drill holes into the table to obtain it. I demand a fountain's unceasing enlivenment. If Maecenas could not sleep without hearing the splashing of a fountain, I cannot eat without it. Do not misunderstand me, I can eat stockfish without it; but I cannot eat at a banquet without it; I can drink water without it, but I cannot drink wine at a banquet without it.**

If the Dane inspires you, perhaps you're a candidate for . . .

The Kierkegaard Diet: "Philosophical Doggerel," personal website, http://members.aol.com/Philosdog/Kierkegaard.html.

MONTAIGNE, MICHEL. "Of Experience." Translated by Charles Cotton. Huafan University website, http://fl.hfu.edu.tw/montaigne/montaigne-essays2.html#XXI.

The art of physic is not so fixed, that we need be without authority for whatever we do; it changes according to climates and moons; according to Fernel and to Scaliger. If your physician does not think it good for you to sleep, to drink wine, or to eat such and such meats, never trouble yourself; I will find you another that shall not be of his opinion; the diversity of medical arguments and opinions embraces all sorts of forms.

NIETZSCHE, FRIEDRICH. *Ecce Homo.* http://users.compaqnet.be/cn127103/Nietzsche_ecce_homo/

I am much more interested in another question on which the "salvation of humanity" depends much more than upon any piece of theological curiosity: the question of nutrition. For ordinary purposes, it may be formulated thus: "How precisely must thou nourish thyself in order to attain to thy maximum of power, or virtue in the Renaissance style of virtue free from moralism?" Here my experiences -have been the worst possible; I am surprised that it took me so long to become aware of this question and to derive "understanding" from my experiences. . . .

In a very enervating climate it is, inadvisable to begin the day with tea: an hour before, it is a good thing to have a cup of thick cocoa, free from oil.

PLATO. *Republic.* Translated by Benjamin Jowett. Masachusetts Institute of Technology website, the Internet Classics Archive, http://classics.mit.edu/Plato/republic.html.

My meaning may be learned from Homer; he, you know, feeds his heroes at their feasts, when they are campaigning, on soldiers' fare; they have no fish, although they are on the shores of the Hellespont, and they are not allowed boiled meats but only roast, which is the food most convenient for soldiers, requiring only that they should light a fire, and not involving the trouble of carrying about pots and pans.

True.

And I can hardly be mistaken in saying that sweet sauces are nowhere mentioned in Homer. In proscribing them, however, he is not singular; all professional athletes are well aware that a man who is to be in good condition should take nothing of the kind.

Yes, he said; and knowing this, they are quite right in not taking them.

ROUSSEAU, JEAN JACQUES. *Emile.* Translated by Grace Roosevelt, Barbara Foxley. Columbia University Institute for Learning Technologies website, http://www.ilt.columbia.edu/pedagogies/rousseau/Contents2.html.

Everything is not food for man, and what may be food for him is not all equally suitable; it depends on the constitution of his species, the climate he lives in, his individual temperament, and the way of living which his condition demands.

We would die of hunger or poison if we had to wait till experience taught us to know and choose food fit for ourselves. But a supreme goodness which has made pleasure the instrument of self-preservation to sentient beings teaches us through our palate what is suitable for our stomach. There is no better doctor than a man's own appetite, and in a state of nature I do not doubt that the food he would find the most agreeable wouldn't also be the most healthy for him.

THOREAU, HENRY DAVID. *Walden.* Pelagus website, http://www.pelagus.org/books/WALDEN,_by_Henry_David_Thoreau_1.html.

The practical objection to animal food in my case was its uncleanness; and besides, when I had caught and cleaned and cooked and eaten my fish, they seemed not to have fed me essentially. It was insignificant and unnecessary, and cost more than it came to. A little bread or a few potatoes would have done as well, with less trouble and filth. Like many of my contemporaries, I had rarely for many years used animal food, or tea, or coffee, &c.; not so much because of any ill effects which I had traced to them, as because they were not agreeable to my imagination. The repugnance to animal food is not the effect of experience, but is an instinct. . . . I believe that every man who has ever been earnest to preserve his higher or poetic faculties in the best condition has been particularly inclined to abstain from animal food, and from much food of any kind.

Nouvelle Cuisine

CURTIN, DEANE and Lisa Heldke, eds. *Cooking, Eating, Thinking: Transformative Philosophies of Food.* Bloomington: Indiana University Press, 1992.

GEORGE, KATHRYN PAXTON. *Animal, Vegetable or Woman: A Feminist Critique of Ethical Vegetarianism.* Stony Brook: State University of New York Press, 2000.

HELDKE, LISA. *Exotic Appetites: Ruminations of a Food Adventurer.* New York: Routledge, 2003.

IGGERS, JEREMY. *The Garden of Eating: Food, Sex and the Hunger for Meaning.* New York: Basic Books, 1996.

KORSMEYER, CAROLYN. *Making Sense of Taste.* Ithaca: Cornell University Press, 1999.

———, ed. *The Taste Culture Reader: Flavor, Food and Meaning* Forthcoming, Berg.

KORTHALS, MICHIEL. *Before Dinner: Philosophy and Ethics of Food.* Dordrecht: Springer, 2004.

MEPHAM, BEN. *Food Ethics.* London: Routledge, 1996.

ONFRAY, MICHEL. *Le Ventre des Philosophes: Critique de la Raison Dietetique.* LGF, 1990.

———. *La Raison Gourmande: Philosophy du Goût.* B. Grasset, 1995.

———. *Les Formes du Temps: theorie du Sauternes.* Diffusion Seuil, 1996.

PROBYN, ELSPETH. *Carnal Appetites: FoodSexIdentities.* London: Routledge, 2000.

REVEL, JEAN-FRANÇOIS. *Culture and Cuisine.* New York: Doubleday, 1982.

SERRES, MICHEL. *The Parasite.* Baltimore: Johns Hopkins University Press, 1982.

TELFER, ELIZABETH. *Food for Thought: Philosophy and Food.* London: Routledge, 1996.

THOMPSON, PAUL. *The Spirit of the Soil.* New York: Routledge, 1995.

WATSON, RICHARD. *The Philosopher's Diet: How to Lose Weight and Change the World.* Boston: Godine, 1999.

Journals

Agriculture and Human Values.

Food, Culture and Society.

Gastronomica.

Journal of Agricultural and Environmental Ethics.

Philosophy Today 31 (2001): Special issue on philosophy and food edited by Jeremy Iggers.

Organizations Exploring Food and Philosophy Issues

Association for the Study of Food and Society
http://www.food-culture.org/

Agriculture, Food and Human Values Association
http://www.clas.ufl.edu/users/rhaynes/afhvs/

Convivium: The Philosophy and Food Roundtable
http://www.gustavus.edu/Groups/convivium/

Dietary Preferences of Contributors

Randall E. Auxier is Professor of Philosophy at Southern Illinois University in the secluded town of Carbondale, where, due to some unfortunate experiments with depleted uranium, boneless chicken breasts now grow on the bushes, allowing him to be the first surviving Atkins vegan, and a thin person of conscience. Randy often sings "Big Rock Candy Mountain" to his colleagues and students, and laments the blight that killed the cigarette trees.

Rebecca Bamford received her Ph.D. in Philosophy from the University of Durham, England, in 2003. She is currently an Andrew Mellon Postdoctoral Research Fellow in Philosophy at Rhodes University, RSA. Her research follows a strict regime of Nietzsche studies, increasingly supplemented by some of the meatier issues in the philosophy of mind and psychology. Rebecca has stuck to a low-starch lifestyle for a number of years, even though it means that her laundry has lots more creases, and found adapting to having less bread easy, because academics don't earn much anyway.

Bat-Ami Bar On is Professor of Philosophy and Women's Studies at Binghamton University (SUNY). Her primary research is on violence. She is the author of *The Subject of Violence: Arendtean Exercises in Understanding* (2002). She has published in feminist anthologies and in *Hypatia*. Her most recent work on terrorism and war appears in the British *Philosopher's Magazine*, the Swedish *ORD&BILD*, and in the *International Feminist Journal of Politics*. She is hoping for the perfect nonfat olive oil to come on the market soon.

Corrinne Bedecarré teaches philosophy at Normandale Community College in the Twin Cities area of Minnesota. Atkins has provided her with just the carte blanche needed to spend her life wallowing in cheese and eggs. Her critique of Atkins supports eating them with enormous quantities of bread. Writing about dieting has increased her hunger for philosophy, feminism, and food.

Marty Bender is a Senior Research Scientist at The Land Institute in Salina, Kansas. He studied the energetics of the institute's Sunshine Farm from 1992 to 2001 and is in the process of writing a book on the project. In his current field research, he is comparing the composting properties of Atkins Quick Quisine ™ Frozen Pasta packaging with that of Ruffles™ Natural Reduced Fat Sea-Salted Potato Chips.

Amy Bentley is an associate professor in the Department of Nutrition, Food Studies, and Public Health at New York University. A cultural historian by training, she is the author of *Eating for Victory: Food Rationing and the Politics of Domesticity* (1998) as well as several articles on food history and culture. Since alternative lifestyles tend to raise hackles, Amy thinks it's only a matter of time before protestors seek a Constitutional amendment to ban the "Atkins lifestyle."

Raymond D. Boisvert teaches at Siena College. Before succumbing to his guilty pleasure, philosophy of food, he produced some real academic books (*Dewey's Metaphysics, John Dewey: Re-Thinking Our Time*). His downfall accelerated with the insight that Descartes should never have said *Cogito, ergo sum,* "I think, therefore I am." It should have been: *Cogito, ergo dim sum,* "I think, therefore let's eat."

Stan Cox is a Senior Research Scientist at The Land Institute in Salina, Kansas. He is a plant breeder working to develop perennial grain crops that will produce food while conserving soil and water. He also writes on environmental and political issues. However, he is a somewhat careless reader; as a result, he has been eating a low-crab diet since 2003. He has lost about ten pounds so far.

Dan Dennis began thinking about philosophy as a teenager, when he was given the job of walking the family dog every night. "Why me?" was his first line of philosophical enquiry, but he soon found himself gazing in wonder at the starlit sky, and trying to find meaning in life. This was subsequently coupled with attempts to solve more difficult and profound questions such as "How can I get a girlfriend?" and "Why do I enjoy chocolate?" He was encouraged by his parents to do a degree in Electronics in order to "get a good job," but his inability to get up before lunchtime marked him out for a career in philosophy. He recently completed a Ph.D. on treating human beings as ends, at Edinburgh University, which seeks to establish firm ethical foundations for harmonious interactions between human beings, and to understand what is truly best for a human being. He is an online philosophy tutor for Oxford University and a selection of his writings can be found at www.pure-ethics.com. Dan tries to make the world a better place than it would have been without him.

DAVID DETMER is Professor of Philosophy at Purdue University Calumet. He is the author of *Sartre Explained* (forthcoming), *Challenging Postmodernism: Philosophy and the Politics of Truth* (2003), and *Freedom as a Value: A Critique of the Ethical Theory of Jean-Paul Sartre* (1988), as well as essays on a variety of philosophical topics. He denounces white flour in all of its forms.

LISA HELDKE writes and teaches pragmatist and feminist philosophy at Gustavus Adolphus College. Previous writings on food and philosophy include the co-edited anthology, *Cooking, Eating, Thinking: Transformative Philosophies of Food*, and the monograph *Exotic Appetites: Ruminations of a Food Adventurer*. She co-edits *Philosophers on Holiday*, a periodic periodical in the philosophical travel-and-leisure genre. (Find it on the web at http://www.gustavus .edu/~poconnor.) Her Atkins credentials include the co-authorship of "St. Cholestera: A Life," the hagiography of the patron saint of butter. She actually thinks *un*sliced bread is the greatest thing since sliced bread.

WILLIAM IRWIN is Associate Professor of Philosophy at King's College, Pennsylvania. He is the author of *Intentionalist Interpretation: A Philosophical Explanation and Defense* and has published articles on aesthetics in leading journals. He has edited *Seinfeld and Philosophy*, *The Simpsons and Philosophy*, *The Matrix and Philosophy*, and *More Matrix and Philosophy*. As a real man—an Atkins man—Bill does not eat quiche, at least not the crust.

CHRISTINE KNIGHT is an off-and-on low-carber, who tends to follow her grilled fish and salad with her favourite spicy plum cake. She is also a Ph.D. student researching socio-cultural aspects of the low-carbohydrate diet trend, and is jointly based at the Discipline of English at the University of Adelaide in South Australia, and the Human Nutrition division of the Commonwealth Scientific and Industrial Research Organisation (CSIRO). Christine's research has provided the perfect excuse to test a multitude of new dietary regimes on friends and family, who consequently now share her obsession with food and nutrition.

Kerri Mommer is a book editor who lives in northwest Indiana and works in Chicago. A linguist by training (Ph.D. in linguistics from Northwestern University), she disputes the common assumption that the phrase *low-carb diet* has Indo-European roots and thinks she may have found evidence that it is derived from *neva-eetagrayn*, a word that means "hunter with 16 percent body fat" in several languages in the Eastern Sudanic sub-family of the Chari-Nilo language family.

Daniel O'Connell is currently completing a doctoral dissertation in philosophy on the notion of "the sight of the mind" (or *visus mentis*) in the writings of the fifteenth-century thinker Nicolaus Cusanus, which will be published in 2006. He is doing so with the aid of a grant from the Fulbright Commission in Berlin, and is a visiting researcher at the Institute for Cusanus-Research at Trier University in Rheinland-Pfalz until February 2006. After a recent trip to Cambridge University for a conference, he would like to echo Brillat-Savarin's third aphorism and say that the destiny of nations does indeed depend on the way in which they are fed and that he, for one, is relieved to be back on the Continent and away from the so-called English breakfast. He lives right in the heart of Old Europe where—through the aid of a (whimsically) modified Atkins diet involving weekly visits to his local butcher and judicious use of the Riesling wines from the Mosel Valley (not to mention the lack of a car)—he has lost more than ten kilos since he moved to Trier last October.

Fabio Parasecoli joyfully commutes between Rome and New York City. After working as a correspondent in foreign affairs and political issues, he concluded that suffering from mild food poisoning is better that dodging bullets in jungles and deserts. This life-changing insight made him shift to food writing. He is now an editor for the Italian magazine *Gambero Rosso*. He helped found the program for Communication and Journalism in Food and Wine at the Città del Gusto School in Rome. He also teaches Food Studies at New York University. He is the author of *Food Culture in Italy* (2004).

Cynthia Pineo, a philosophy book editor in Chicago, has been pondering the following Atkins-related conundrum: If you deconstruct your sandwich and don't eat the bread, is it still a sandwich? To avoid the dilemma, she recommends ordering a low-carb wrap instead (rubbery texture, but not unpleasantly so).

David Ramsay Steele is the author of *From Marx to Mises* (1992) and co-author (with Michael R. Edelstein) of *Three Minute Therapy* (1997). His writings have appeared in such unlikely places as *Ethics*, *Liberty*,

International Philosophical Quarterly, and *National Review*. He is a contributor to the forthcoming *New Encyclopedia of Unbelief*. Dr. Steele has advanced the theory that cheesecake contains a little-known enzyme guaranteeing rapid weight loss. When pressed, he points out that this assertion is the expression of a profound spiritual truth about the human condition and is therefore beyond the reach of one-dimensional bourgeois-positivist "testing."

ABBY WILKERSON, a philosopher, lives in Riverdale (yes, where Nancy Drew ate platefuls of sandwiches with her chums), Maryland, and teaches in the University Writing Program at George Washington University in Washington, D.C. She is the author of *Diagnosis—Difference: The Moral Authority of Medicine* (1998). Early training as a vegetarian in West Texas, where even the vegetables come with meat, conditioned her instinctive rejection of the Atkins diet.

CATHERINE A. WOMACK is Assistant Professor of Philosophy at Bridgewater State College in Massachusetts. Her primary areas of research are philosophy of mathematics and science; she has published articles in various journals and conference proceedings. In the past year her work has combined the personal and the philosophical: she has been doing research on a project on causality and obesity and has also lost fifty-five pounds. She would love to write her own diet book, but has not yet figured out how to extend the advice "eat less and exercise more" to 150 pages.

Glycemic Index